ANNALS *of* THE NEW YORK ACADEMY OF SCIENCES

VOLUME 1284

ISBN-10: 1-57331-895-7; **ISBN-13:** 978-1-57331-895-2

ISSUE

The Renaissance of Cancer Immunotherapy

The 7th International Cancer Vaccine Symposium

ISSUE EDITORS

Olivera J. Finn[a] and Gerold Schuler[b]

[a]University of Pittsburgh and [b]University Hospital of Erlangen

T0344668

TABLE OF CONTENTS

Annals of the New York Academy of Sciences (ISSN: 0077-8923 [print]; ISSN: 1749-6632 [online]) is published 30 times a year on behalf of the New York Academy of Sciences by Wiley Subscription Services, Inc., a Wiley Company, 111 River Street, Hoboken, NJ 07030-5774.

Mailing: *Annals of the New York Academy of Sciences* is mailed standard rate.

Postmaster: Send all address changes to ANNALS OF THE NEW YORK ACADEMY OF SCIENCES, Journal Customer Services, John Wiley & Sons Inc., 350 Main Street, Malden, MA 02148-5020.

Disclaimer: The publisher, the New York Academy of Sciences, and the editors cannot be held responsible for errors or any consequences arising from the use of information contained in this publication; the views and opinions expressed do not necessarily reflect those of the publisher, the New York Academy of Sciences, and editors, neither does the publication of advertisements constitute any endorsement by the publisher, the New York Academy of Sciences and editors of the products advertised.

Publisher: *Annals of the New York Academy of Sciences* is published by Wiley Periodicals, Inc., Commerce Place, 350 Main Street, Malden, MA 02148; Telephone: 781 388 8200; Fax: 781 388 8210.

Journal Customer Services: For ordering information, claims, and any inquiry concerning your subscription, please go to www.wileycustomerhelp.com/ask or contact your nearest office. *Americas:* Email: cs-journals@wiley.com; Tel:+1 781 388 8598 or 1 800 835 6770 (Toll free in the USA & Canada). *Europe, Middle East, Asia:* Email: cs-journals@wiley. com; Tel: +44 (0) 1865 778315. *Asia Pacific:* Email: cs-journals@wiley.com; Tel: +65 6511 8000. *Japan:* For Japanese speaking support, Email: cs-japan@wiley.com; Tel: +65 6511 8010 or Tel (toll-free): 005 316 50 480. Visit our Online Customer Get-Help available in 6 languages at www.wileycustomerhelp.com.

Information for Subscribers: *Annals of the New York Academy of Sciences* is published in 30 volumes per year. Subscription prices for 2013 are: Print & Online: US$6,053 (US), US$6,589 (Rest of World), €4,269 (Europe), £3,364 (UK). Prices are exclusive of tax. Australian GST, Canadian GST, and European VAT will be applied at the appropriate rates. For more information on current tax rates, please go to www.wileyonlinelibrary.com/tax-vat. The price includes online access to the current and all online back files to January 1, 2009, where available. For other pricing options, including access information and terms and conditions, please visit www.wileyonlinelibrary.com/access.

Delivery Terms and Legal Title: Where the subscription price includes print volumes and delivery is to the recipient's address, delivery terms are Delivered at Place (DAP); the recipient is responsible for paying any import duty or taxes. Title to all volumes transfers FOB our shipping point, freight prepaid. We will endeavour to fulfill claims for missing or damaged copies within six months of publication, within our reasonable discretion and subject to availability.

Back issues: Recent single volumes are available to institutions at the current single volume price from cs-journals@wiley.com. Earlier volumes may be obtained from Periodicals Service Company, 11 Main Street, Germantown, NY 12526, USA. Tel: +1 518 537 4700, Fax: +1 518 537 5899, Email: psc@periodicals.com. For submission instructions, subscription, and all other information visit: www.wileyonlinelibrary.com/journal/nyas.

Production Editors: Kelly McSweeney and Allie Struzik (email: nyas@wiley.com).

Commercial Reprints: Dan Nicholas (email: dnicholas@wiley.com).

Membership information: Members may order copies of *Annals* volumes directly from the Academy by visiting www. nyas.org/annals, emailing customerservice@nyas.org, faxing +1 212 298 3650, or calling 1 800 843 6927 (toll free in the USA), or +1 212 298 8640. For more information on becoming a member of the New York Academy of Sciences, please visit www.nyas.org/membership. Claims and inquiries on member orders should be directed to the Academy at email: membership@nyas.org or Tel: 1 800 843 6927 (toll free in the USA) or +1 212 298 8640.

Printed in the USA by The Sheridan Group.

View *Annals* online at www.wileyonlinelibrary.com/journal/nyas.

Abstracting and Indexing Services: *Annals of the New York Academy of Sciences* is indexed by MEDLINE, Science Citation Index, and SCOPUS. For a complete list of A&I services, please visit the journal homepage at www. wileyonlinelibrary.com/journal/nyas.

Access to *Annals* is available free online within institutions in the developing world through the AGORA initiative with the FAO, the HINARI initiative with the WHO, and the OARE initiative with UNEP. For information, visit www. aginternetwork.org, www.healthinternetwork.org, www.oarescience.org.

Annals of the New York Academy of Sciences accepts articles for Open Access publication. Please visit http://olabout.wiley.com/WileyCDA/Section/id-406241.html for further information about OnlineOpen.

Wiley's Corporate Citizenship initiative seeks to address the environmental, social, economic, and ethical challenges faced in our business and which are important to our diverse stakeholder groups. Since launching the initiative, we have focused on sharing our content with those in need, enhancing community philanthropy, reducing our carbon impact, creating global guidelines and best practices for paper use, establishing a vendor code of ethics, and engaging our colleagues and other stakeholders in our efforts. Follow our progress at www.wiley.com/go/citizenship.

Ann. N.Y. Acad. Sci. ISSN 0077-8923

Introduction to *The Renaissance of Cancer Immunotherapy*

On September 9–11, 2012, in Florence, Italy, the Hasumi International Research Foundation sponsored the conference "Renaissance of Cancer Immunotherapy," the seventh in a series of international symposia on cancer vaccines (the International Cancer Vaccine Symposium (ICVS)). Both the title and the location were chosen with the specific intent of acknowledging the long, winding, and arduous road traveled by cancer immunologists. The "dark ages," when, in spite of evidence to the contrary, the immune system was not considered in any way involved with cancer, has been replaced by the age of acceptance and reawakening—the renaissance of the idea that the immune system is among the most important, if not the most important, player in cancer development. Knowledge accumulated over the last several decades has elucidated, down to molecular detail, the functions of the immune system during cancer development, and, most importantly, it has given rise to immunotherapeutic approaches that are positively influencing clinical outcome for cancer patients. Just in the period between the 6th ICVS, held in 2008 at the New York Academy of Sciences in New York City, and the one in Florence in 2012, a therapeutic cancer vaccine for prostate cancer has been approved, as have been several therapeutic antibodies that target cancer directly or target the immune system to enhance its anticancer effects.

The Hasumi International Research Foundation is inextricably linked with the long history of cancer immunotherapy. Dr. Kiichiro Hasumi, working at the turn of the last century, was interested in determining the origins of cancer, and in 1931 he theorized that viruses cause cancers, a revolutionary theory that was not readily accepted by the scientific establishment of that time. Modern science has since obtained proof of the viral origin of a number of human cancer types, including hepatocellular carcinoma being caused by hepatitis B virus (HBV), cervical and oral cancer by human papillomavirus (HPV), Burkitt's lymphoma by Epstein–Barr virus (EBV), Kaposi sarcoma by KSHV, and one form of skin cancer by Merkel cell virus. There will undoubtedly be additional cancer-causing viruses discovered. Vaccines against infections with such viruses, as has been shown for EBV and more recently for HPV, will prevent those cancers from occurring and in some cases help in their cure. Without the benefit of the knowledge of individual viruses, Dr. Hasumi correctly hypothesized that cancer cells would carry viral antigens and that a vaccine composed of cancer cells themselves would immunize against relevant but unknown viral antigens and stimulate the immune system to recognize the cancer. Thus he created the Hasumi vaccine, which was first tested in 1931. In 1946, he established the Electro-Chemical & Cancer Institute responsible for producing vaccines for individual patients, and in 1948 he opened the Shukokai Clinic in Tokyo where patients were treated. Cancer immunotherapy as initially practiced in the clinic by Dr. Kiichiro Hasumi used only the Hasumi vaccine, but as new knowledge accumulated, and as additional immunotherapeutic approaches were developed around the world, the clinic's mission to apply immunotherapy to cancer patients was broadened to include additional immune-based therapies. This expended mission was undertaken and promoted by his son, Dr. Kenichiro Hasumi.

In the last 50 years, over 100,000 cancer patients in Japan and from around the world have been treated with the Hasumi vaccine, and in the most recent years many have also received dendritic cell–based vaccines or adoptive therapy with activated cytotoxic T cells or lymphokine-activated killer cells. In 1999,

doi: 10.1111/nyas.12153

v

Dr. Kenichiro Hasumi established the Hasumi International Research Foundation dedicated to fostering communication among cancer immunologists and immunotherapists around the world with the goal of speeding up scientific progress in the laboratory and developing immunotherapy in the clinic.

Almost a century after Dr. Kiichiro Hasumi contemplated viral antigens as specific tumor antigens and worked on personalized cancer vaccines based on the patient's own tumor, technological advances are now allowing genetic profiling of each patient's tumor, again suggesting an individualized approach to cancer vaccines. A number of modern-day therapeutic cancer vaccines are based on an individual patient's killed tumor cells, tumor cell mRNA, tumor cell lysates, or known mutated tumor proteins. For preventive cancer vaccines, the choices are the known viral antigens, commonly mutated proteins, or other antigens shared among tumors of many individuals.

What early cancer vaccinologists like Dr. Hasumi did not know were the details of the complex interactions between the immune system and cancer that affected the ability of the patient to respond to cancer vaccines. That knowledge, more than the type of a vaccine or the choice of the antigens, is changing the field of cancer immunotherapy. Previous failures of immunotherapy contributed to the discovery of many mechanisms that suppress the immune system and make it refractory to attempts to stimulate its anticancer function through immunotherapy. Even passive immunotherapy, such as infusion of anticancer antibodies, is now known to be compromised by the suppressed immune system that cannot contribute to the effector function of these antibodies. Knowing the state of the patient's immune system and the specific functions that are either enhanced or compromised by the presence of cancer supports the design of combination therapies intended to target both the cancer and the immune system to achieve a curative environment in the patient.

This new era of cancer immunotherapy was fully represented at the meeting by the speakers, who are the leaders in this field. For two days and within six sessions that covered the tumor microenvironment and antitumor immunity, cell-based anticancer vaccines, peptide-based anticancer vaccines, understanding and enhancing spontaneous antitumor immunity, antitumor immunity through the lens of systems biology, and progress on the path to translation to the clinic, the newest observations were shared and the paths toward more successful immunotherapy were proposed. Examples of the work discussed can be found in the short reviews we have collected for this volume.

The 7th ICVS had another important goal: to commemorate the contributions to the field of cancer vaccines, and vaccines in general, of the late Ralph M. Steinman, M.D., 2011 Nobel Laureate in Physiology or Medicine, for his discovery of dendritic cells. The symposium was held on the first anniversary of his death.

Ralph Steinman always considered the physiological context of scientific findings, and he was very much convinced that it is our duty to help translate them into the clinic to advance diagnosis and therapy of diseases. This attitude, likely fostered by his clinical training as a physician, was reflected in what he said and did. Early on he tellingly referred to dendritic cells (DCs) as *nature's adjuvant* and began to emphasize that we must learn to harness the biology of DCs to modulate the immune system and influence diseases, either by enhancing (in infections and cancer) or dampening (in transplantation, autoimmunity, and allergy) antigen-specific T cell responses.

Ralph always emphasized that prophylactic vaccination against infection, which is based on the induction of neutralizing antibodies, is the fascinating success story of immunology, yet the huge potential of T cell–based vaccination has yet to be realized. His wish was to help build better T cell–based vaccines, and he achieved this not only through his scientific findings but also by passionately teaching young colleagues and supporting them along their career as well as by inspiring other scientists and convincing them that understanding DC biology was important for vaccine development. He also felt that *in vitro* and preclinical mouse experiments, although informative, must be confirmed by studies in humans as quickly as possible. He was well aware that organizing, financing, and performing clinical trials is often demanding and that the merits are frequently modest because the mechanistic workup and insight from a single human study cannot be compared to simpler experimental systems, including studies in mice. This led to an editorial in the *Journal of Experimental Medicine* (JEM) in 2003, by Ralph, who was at that time one of the JEM editors, encouraging the submission of manuscripts that would report research in human subjects. Only two years later, Ralph was able to write another editorial reporting the success of this initiative that showed a large increase of submission of such manuscripts, and where he also shared his valuable insights on the research in human subjects.

Whenever possible Ralph tried to convince scientists and decision makers that the field of immunotherapy holds enormous potential not only for better understanding how the human immune system and body work, but also for providing new and better approaches for fighting cancer and other diseases. He made it clear that basic research directly in humans was an absolute necessity and that experimental medicine in humans is underdeveloped primarily because of organizational problems and inappropriate funding mechanisms. His participation in the discussions with the European Commission (EC) in Brussels, for example, was crucial for the successful establishment and EC funding of initiatives such as Dendritic Cells for Novel Immunotherapies (DC-THERA) focusing on DC-based vaccination against cancer.

Early on Ralph Steinman had developed the hypothesis that tumor immunity is not effectively induced in tumor-bearing hosts due to the lack of tumor antigen presentation by mature immunogenic DCs *in vivo*, a problem that could be circumvented by delivering tumor antigens on autologous mature DCs, that is, DC vaccination. Adoptively transferred DCs isolated from the mouse spleen could indeed induce immunity and in certain tumor models also induce clinical effects. In humans, DCs enriched from blood and used in a vaccine showed effects in B cell lymphomas. Many DC-based vaccines were tested; and in 2010 the Dendreon Corporation received FDA approval for its DC-based vaccine Provenge® for the treatment of castration-resistant metastatic prostate cancer. Each dose of this vaccine must, however, be generated from a separate apheresis by preparing a low-density fraction, which is enriched in DCs, as Ralph Steinman´s group had demonstrated when first describing human DCs in blood, followed by incubating it with a PAP-GM-CSF fusion protein. Ralph was closely involved with the first use of DC-based vaccines in patients with melanoma and multiple myeloma.

In his last extensive review (Decisions about dendritic cells: past, present, and future. 2012. *Annu. Rev. Immunol.* **30**: 1–22), Ralph delineated his second entry, the vast realm of vaccines, by targeting antigens to DCs *in vivo* through the use of antibodies specific for C-type lectins expressed on the surface of DCs, in conjunction with a suitable maturation stimulus to induce robust immunity. This promising approach is being actively pursued by many of his colleagues.

The field of cancer immunotherapy and vaccines has lost an important driving force and an inspiring leader. Ralph M. Steinman´s scientific lifework paved the way for developing better vaccines not only because of his seminal basic science discoveries, but also because if his own commitment and contributions to translational medicine. His lasting influence on cancer immunotherapy was obvious in the presentations given by the speakers of the 7th International Cancer Vaccine Symposium in Florence and permeates the reviews selected for this volume.

Olivera J. Finn
University of Pittsburgh
Pittsburgh, Pennsylvania

Gerold Schuler
University Hospital of Erlangen
Erlangen, Germany

Ann. N.Y. Acad. Sci. ISSN 0077-8923

ANNALS OF THE NEW YORK ACADEMY OF SCIENCES
Issue: *The Renaissance of Cancer Immunotherapy*

Cancer immunoediting: antigens, mechanisms, and implications to cancer immunotherapy

Matthew D. Vesely and Robert D. Schreiber

Department of Pathology and Immunology, Washington University School of Medicine, St. Louis, Missouri

Address for correspondence: Robert D. Schreiber, Department of Pathology and Immunology, Washington University School of Medicine, 660 South Euclid Avenue, St. Louis, MO 63110. schreiber@immunology.wustl.edu

Accumulated data from animal models and human cancer patients strongly support the concept that the immune system can identify and control nascent tumor cells in a process called cancer immunosurveillance. In addition, the immune system can also promote tumor progression through chronic inflammation, immunoselection of poorly immunogenic variants, and suppressing antitumor immunity. Together, the dual host-protective and tumor-promoting actions of immunity are referred to as cancer immunoediting. The current framework of cancer immunoediting is a dynamic process comprised of three distinct phases: elimination, equilibrium, and escape. Recently, we demonstrated that immunoselection by CD8+ T cells of tumor variants lacking strong tumor-specific antigens represents one mechanism by which cancer cells escape tumor immunity and points toward the future of personalized cancer therapy.

Keywords: cancer immunoediting; immunosurveillance; tumor antigens; immunotherapy; tumor escape; cancer genome

Introduction

Cancer immunoediting

A plethora of evidence now provides strong support for cancer immunoediting, a process wherein immunity functions not only as an extrinsic tumor suppressor but also to shape tumor immunogenicity.[1] In its most complex form, cancer immunoediting occurs in three sequential phases: elimination, equilibrium, and escape. Elimination is a modern view of the older notion of cancer immunosurveillance, in which innate and adaptive immunity work together to detect and destroy transformed cells long before they become clinically apparent. However, sometimes tumor cell variants may not be completely eliminated but instead enter into an equilibrium phase in which the immune system controls net tumor cell outgrowth; in this phase, adaptive immunity constrains the growth of clinically undetectable occult tumor cells and edits tumor cell immunogenicity.[2] Finally, the functional dormancy of the tumor cell population may be broken, leading to progression of the cells into the escape phase, during which edited tumors of reduced immunogenicity begin to grow progressively in an immunologically unrestrained manner, establish an immunosuppressive tumor microenvironment, and eventually become clinically apparent.[3] Importantly, escape from immune control is now acknowledged to be one of the hallmarks of cancer.[4]

The antigens of unedited tumors

A central tenet of tumor immunology in general, and the cancer immunoediting process in particular, is that tumor cells express antigens that distinguish them from their nontransformed counterparts, thus permitting their recognition by T cells and their eventual destruction by immunological mechanisms. Although a deep understanding of human and mouse tumor antigens currently exists, it comes nearly entirely from analyses of tumor cells derived from immunocompetent hosts, which were likely subjected to the sculpting forces of cancer immunoediting during their development. Little is known about the antigens expressed in nascent tumor cells, for example, whether they are sufficient

doi: 10.1111/nyas.12105
Ann. N.Y. Acad. Sci. 1284 (2013) 1–5 © 2013 New York Academy of Sciences.

to induce host-protective, antitumor immune responses, or whether their expression is modulated by the immune system.

We realized that such questions might be answered by defining the antigens expressed in unedited sarcoma cell lines derived from 3'-methylcholanthrene (MCA)–treated, immunodeficient $Rag2^{-/-}$ mice because such induced tumor cells phenotypically resemble highly immunogenic, nascent, primary tumor cells.[5] However, current methods to identify tumor antigens using expression-cloning approaches are time and effort intensive, and are not well suited to establishing a tumor's antigenic landscape. Recent advances in genome sequencing have made possible rapid and cost effective methods to define cancer genomes, and have established that, while they acquire some mutations involved in the transformation process (*driver* mutations), cancer cells also develop many *passenger* mutations, in part, as a consequence of the genomic instability that is a characteristic of transformed cells. It has been proposed that some of these mutations result in the expression of tumor-specific proteins that are, in turn, tumor-specific antigens for T cells.[6] However, until recently, this had not been experimentally demonstrated.

Recent work from our laboratory[7] used a novel form of exome sequencing (cDNA capture sequencing or cDNA CapSeq) to define the mutational profile of two independent, unedited MCA sarcomas (d42m1 and H31m1). By pipelining the sequencing data for one of these tumors (d42m1) into major histocompatibility complex (MHC) class I epitope prediction algorithms, we identified a potential mutational antigen of the unedited d42m1 cells, validated its identity as the major rejection antigen using expression cloning techniques, and showed that antigen loss via a T cell–dependent immunoselection process represents the mechanism underlying cancer immunoediting of this tumor. This study[7] thus provides mechanistic insights into the process of cancer immunoediting and points to the future potential that cancer genome analysis may have on the fields of tumor immunology and cancer immunotherapy.

Cancer genome sequencing and antigen discovery

Using cDNA CapSeq, we identified 3,737 nonsynonymous mutations in d42m1 cells and 2,677 non-synonymous mutations in H31m1 cells. However, only 5% of the mutations were shared between d42m1 and H31m1, which explains the unique immunogenicity that each cell line displays. Interestingly, both d42m1 and H31m1 had activating mutations in codon 12 of the *Kras* proto-oncogene and inactivating mutations in the tumor suppressor gene *Trp53*. When comparing the sequence data of d42m1 and H31m1 sarcoma cells to those of human cancer genomes, we found that the former most closely resemble genomes of carcinogen-induced lung cancers from smokers in both the number and type of mutations (e.g., C/A or G/T transversions).

Thus, cancer exome sequencing of d42m1 and H31m1 cells demonstrated a carcinogen signature similar to that found in lung cancer cells from smokers, but distinct from other human cancers. This raises the possibility that a similar discovery approach may be used to find tumor-specific antigens in human lung cancer.

d42m1 tumor variants

The d42m1 sarcoma cell line displays a sporadic tendency to produce escape tumors following transplantation into naive, syngeneic wild-type mice. Furthermore, cell lines derived from escape tumors of parental d42m1 (d42m1-es1, d42m1-es2, and d42m1-es3) consistently formed progressively growing tumors when transplanted into naive syngeneic recipients. Thus, unedited d42m1 tumor cells can undergo immunoediting when transplanted into wild-type mice. The heterogeneous behavior of d42m1 tumor cells in naive immunocompetent mice is due to the parental d42m1 cell line consisting of a disproportionate (80:20) mixture of regressor and progressor tumor cell clones.

Identifying potential d42m1 tumor antigens from genomic data

To identify tumor-specific antigens for CD8$^+$ T cells, we used the data from the cancer exome mutational analysis to identify the antigenic targets of d42m1-specific CD8$^+$ cytotoxic T lymphocytes (CTLs). First, we assessed the theoretical capacity of peptides containing each missense mutation to bind to MHC class I proteins (i.e., to function as neoantigens) by *in silico* analysis. Second, we used a d42m1-specific CD8$^+$ CTL clone derived from a wild-type mouse that had rejected parental d42m1 tumor cells to assess tumor reactivity *in vitro*; the readout of CTL activity against the tumor cells was IFN-γ production by the CD8$^+$ T cells. The d42m1-specific C3 CTL clone was stimulated by parental d42m1 tumor cells and with all regressor d42m1 tumor cell variants, but it was not stimulated by progressor d42m1 tumor cell variants or unrelated MCA sarcoma cells. These results revealed that regressor d42m1 tumor cells share a common rejection antigen. We therefore focused on the limited number of epitopes common to all d42m1 regressor variants. And, together with the fact that recognition of all d42m1 regressor variants by the CTL clone was restricted by H-2D^b, we predicted that an R913L mutation in spectrin-β2 represented the most likely rejection antigen candidate because of its high affinity for H-2D^b.

Next, we established that C3 CTL cells could discriminate between the mutant and wild-type spectrin-β2 peptide sequence 905–913 when presented on H-2D^b. To document that the anti-R913L spectrin-β2 response occurred under physiologic conditions, we used labeled H-2D^b tetramers carrying the mutant spectrin-β2 905–913 peptide to identify tumor antigen–specific CD8$^+$ T cells in d42m1 tumors. Mutant spectrin-β2–specific CD8$^+$ T cells were detected in parental d42m1 tumors and draining lymph nodes, and increased in numbers to peak values just prior to tumor rejection. In contrast, no mutant spectrin-β2–specific CD8$^+$ T cells were detected in d42m1-es3 tumors. These data demonstrate that a mutated gene expressed selectively in unedited d42m1 tumor cells gives rise to a mutant protein that evokes a naturally occurring T cell response in naive wild-type mice. Thus, mutant spectrin-β2 is a genuine tumor-specific antigen of d42m1 sarcoma cells.

Mutant spectrin-β2 is the major rejection antigen of d42m1 tumor cells

To explore whether mutant spectrin-β2 represented the major rejection antigen of parental d42m1 tumor cells, we enforced expression of either the mutant or wild-type forms of spectrin-β2 into cells of one of the d42m1 escape variants, d42m1-es3. When injected into wild-type mice, d42m1-es3 tumor cell clones expressing wild-type spectrin-β2 grew progressively and displayed similar growth kinetics to the parental d42m1-es3 cell line. In contrast, d42m1-es3 tumor cell clones expressing mutant spectrin-β2 were rejected in wild-type but not $Rag2^{-/-}$ mice. Furthermore, CD8$^+$ T cells specific for mutant spectrin-β2 were detected by tetramer

staining of d42m1-es3 tumors that had been reconstituted with mutant spectrin-β2. These results demonstrate that expression of mutant spectrin-β2 is both necessary and sufficient for the rejection of d42m1 tumors, and thus validate it as a major rejection antigen of d42m1 sarcoma cells.

Immunoselection is the immunoediting mechanism for d42m1 tumor cells

Next, we formulated the hypothesis that T cell–dependent immunoselection was a likely mechanism favoring outgrowth of tumor variants that lack strong rejection antigens. This possibility is consistent with our finding that every d42m1 clone that expresses mutant spectrin-β2 was rejected, whereas every clone or variant that lacks mutant spectrin-β2 formed progressively growing tumors. To formally test this hypothesis, we assessed the *in vivo* behavior of a disproportionate mixture of cells consisting of a majority of highly immunogenic d42m1 tumor cells expressing mutant spectrin-β2 (i.e., d42m1-T2) and a minority of a d42m1 tumor cell clone lacking mutant spectrin-β2 (i.e., d42m1-T3). When this mixture was transplanted into wild-type mice, 5 of 20 (25%) developed escape tumors, a result that closely resembles what was observed with parental d42m1 tumor cells in wild-type recipients. Furthermore, tumors that grew out in wild-type mice consisted of 98% d42m1-T3 tumor cells and lacked mutant spectrin-β2. Thus, escape variants of parental d42m1 tumor cells develop as a consequence of a T cell–dependent immunoselection process that favors the outgrowth of tumor cell clones lacking the major rejection antigen.

For d42m1 tumor cells, we show that an immunoselection process acting on an oligoclonal parental tumor cell population leads to the outgrowth of tumor cell variants that lack the major tumor rejection antigen, in this case, mutant spectrin-β2. The immunoselection that occurs upon exposure to an intact immune system is dependent on adaptive immunity since neither parental d42m1 tumor cells nor the mixture of regressor and progressor d42m1 tumor cell clones undergoes editing when passed through $Rag2^{-/-}$ mice; yet they are edited following transplantation into immunocompetent wild-type mice. Thus, in the case of d42m1, the target of the immunoselection process has been clearly identified as a major rejection antigen. However, this finding does not rule out the possibility that similar immunoediting mechanisms might select for mutations in critical components of the MHC class I antigen processing and presentation pathway, such as the class I heavy chain,[3] β2 microglobulin, or components of IFN-γ receptor signaling,[1] all of which are known to regulate tumor cell recognition by tumor specific CD8[+] T cells.

Personalized immunotherapy and genomics: the antigen landscape

Recent advances in genome sequencing have resulted in unprecedented opportunities to assess genetic influences on disease development. For cancer, most genome sequencing studies have focused on identifying new driver mutations that promote neoplastic development and metastasis, in the hope of obtaining insights that lead to novel cancer-targeted therapeutics or that provide prognostic value.[8] However, we have shown that this same technology, when combined with an *in silico* epitope prediction algorithm, can be used to identify expressed mutations in cancer cells that result in expression of tumor-specific antigens that can be targets for immune-mediated elimination. We predict that this approach may not only provide new insights into basic mechanisms underlying cancer immunoediting but also new opportunities for individualized cancer immunotherapy.

The large datasets of information from the many cancer genome initiatives could be of value to tumor immunologists for defining the antigen landscape—as opposed to the mutational landscape—of human cancers.[9] One application of this approach is that it could be used to identify the subset of cancer patients whose tumors express antigens that may be better targeted by immunotherapy. For example, only about 25% of patients treated with anti-CTLA-4 respond positively, and the reasons for this limited response remain unknown. We suggest that patients who respond to checkpoint blockade immunotherapy may have more immunogenic, tumor-specific mutations, and that these antigens can be identified using cancer exome sequencing and high-throughput bioinformatics; in other words, the genomics approach may provide a mechanism to stratify those patients who would benefit most from this type of therapy. A second application of this approach may provide a mechanism to longitudinally evaluate changes in a tumor's antigenic profile as a consequence of ongoing immunotherapy.

A third application is the rapid identification of the most immunogenic epitopes within a tumor, with the goal of developing personalized cancer vaccines for patients.

It is difficult to predict whether this type of analysis will yield prognostic value in the clinic, as genome analysis can be costly and requires streamlined computational analysis. Nevertheless, third-generation sequencing technologies are already commercially available, and costs for cancer genome sequencing have already started to fall sharply and are likely to continue dropping over the next decade. It should thus be feasible to routinely perform this type of genomic analysis on individual patient's cancer cells in the not-too-distant future.

Remaining questions

Our recent study[7] demonstrates that immunoediting of a tumor results from T cell–dependent immunoselection for tumor cell variants that fail to express highly antigenic mutations. These results not only provide definitive evidence for at least one mechanism underlying the cancer immunoediting process, but also demonstrate the key role that tumor-specific mutations play in the development of a tumor's immunogenic phenotype and subsequent fate.

It is interesting that a single mutant protein manifests such immunodominance as d42m1 tumor cells, an immunodominance that in some ways resembles the immunodominance of certain viral antigens. Many factors may contribute to the immunodominance of mutant spectrin-β2. On the basis of *in silico* analysis, the mutant 905–913 sequence is predicted to interact with H-2D[b] with very high affinity in contrast to the corresponding wild-type sequence, which is predicted to bind only weakly. However, several other factors may also contribute to the immunodominance of mutant spectrin-β2, including antigen abundance, antigen cross presentability, T cell repertoire, or presence of epitopes recognized by regulatory T cells. Clearly, more work is needed to refine the capacity to accurately predict the antigenicity of a mutated protein.

It is unclear from our work whether the mechanism of cellular transformation influences the types of antigens that are eventually expressed by cancer cells. In our model, sarcomas generated from chemical carcinogens are most similar, in the number and type of mutations, to carcinogen-induced human cancers, such as lung cancers from smokers. For the past six decades, the MCA sarcoma system has been an experimental workhorse for tumor immunologists. This may be due to the carcinogen's ability to generate a large number of passenger mutations, which allows for a greater number of potential neoantigens to form that may be recognized by the immune system. We speculate that oncogene-driven models of cancer, which harbor fewer passenger mutations than spontaneous cancers, may not be as readily eradicated or controlled by antitumor immunity. However, in a companion study to ours, Michel DuPage and Tyler Jacks *et al.* demonstrated a key role of dominant antigens in the cancer immunoediting process by using a sarcoma model driven by *Kras* activation and *Trp53* inactivation.[10]

Summary and conclusions

The recent revolution in genomics represents a significant transition in the evolution of the cancer immunoediting concept. In the past, efforts were mostly centered on demonstrating that the process occurs, identifying the key players in it, and attempting to define the positions that they play. Work in this area now enters a new phase in which researchers can begin to elucidate the molecular mechanisms that drive the process, and determine the quality and quantity of tumor antigens expressed in nascently transformed cells that drive immune-mediated elimination and/or sculpting.

The approach of exome sequencing, *in silico* analysis, and CD8$^+$ T cell cloning are beneficial to both basic and clinical scientists. By defining the specific antigenic targets in cancer cells, new levels of understanding of host responses to tumors during ongoing therapy can be obtained. This, in turn, should facilitate the development of new therapeutic opportunities that direct the power and specificity of the immune system to control, and/or destroy, cancer. It may also be useful for identifying subsets of cancer patients whose tumors express antigens that can be most effectively targeted by check-point blockade immunotherapy, and may provide a mechanism to longitudinally evaluate changes in a tumor's antigenic profile as a consequence of ongoing immunotherapy. Therefore, we predict that a genomic approach to tumor antigen identification may, in the future, facilitate the development of individualized cancer immunotherapies directed at tumor-specific—rather than simply cancer-associated—antigens.

Acknowledgments

This work was supported by grants to R.D.S. from the National Cancer Institute, the Ludwig Institute for Cancer Research, the Cancer Research Institute, and the WWWW Foundation. M.D.V. is supported by a predoctoral fellowship from the Cancer Research Institute.

Conflicts of interest

The authors declare no conflicts of interest.

References

1. Vesely, M.D. *et al.* 2011. Natural innate and adaptive immunity to cancer. *Annu. Rev. Immunol.* **29:** 235–271.
2. Koebel, C.M. *et al.* 2007. Adaptive immunity maintains occult cancer in an equilibrium state. *Nature* **450:** 903–907.
3. Khong, H.T. & N.P. Restifo. 2002. Natural selection of tumor variants in the generation of "tumor escape" phenotypes. *Nat. Immunol.* **3:** 999–1005.
4. Hanahan, D. & R.A. Weinberg. 2011. Hallmarks of cancer: the next generation. *Cell* **144:** 646–674.
5. Shankaran, V. *et al.* 2001. IFNγ and lymphocytes prevent primary tumour development and shape tumour immunogenicity. *Nature* **410:** 1107–1111.
6. Segal, N.H. *et al.* 2008. Epitope landscape in breast and colorectal cancer. *Cancer Res.* **68:** 889–892.
7. Matsushita, H. *et al.* 2012. Cancer exome analysis reveals a T-cell-dependent mechanism of cancer immunoediting. *Nature* **482:** 400–404.
8. Stratton, M.R. 2011. Exploring the genomes of cancer cells: progress and promise. *Science* **331:** 1553–1558.
9. Wood, L.D. *et al.* 2007. The genomic landscapes of human breast and colorectal cancers. *Science* **318:** 1108–1113.
10. DuPage, M. *et al.* 2012. Expression of tumour-specific antigens underlies cancer immunoediting. *Nature* **482:** 405–409.

Ann. N.Y. Acad. Sci. ISSN 0077-8923

ANNALS OF THE NEW YORK ACADEMY OF SCIENCES
Issue: *The Renaissance of Cancer Immunotherapy*

Cell-extrinsic effects of the tumor unfolded protein response on myeloid cells and T cells

Maurizio Zanetti

The Laboratory of Immunology, Department of Medicine and Moores Cancer Center, University of California, San Diego, California

Address for correspondence: Maurizio Zanetti, The Laboratory of Immunology, Department of Medicine and Moores Cancer Center, University of California, San Diego, 9500 Gilman Drive, La Jolla, CA 92093-0815. mzanetti@ucsd.edu

Tumor-infiltrating myeloid cells, macrophages, and dendritic cells (DCs) are key regulators of tumor immunity and growth. The origin of tumor-derived signals that instruct myeloid cells in the tumor microenvironment is only partially understood. The endoplasmic reticulum (ER) stress response, or unfolded protein response (UPR), provides survival advantages to tumor growth. However, the cell-extrinsic effects of the tumor UPR on immune cells have not been explored. Our laboratory recently showed that the tumor UPR can be transmitted by yet unidentified factor(s) to myeloid cells, macrophages, and DCs. ER stress transmission to receiver myeloid cells upregulates the production of proinflammatory cytokines, and contextually of arginase I, leading to a proinflammatory/suppressive phenotype. DCs imprinted by tumor-borne ER stress transmissible factor(s) have decreased cross-presentation of antigen and defective cross-priming, causing T cell activation without proliferation. When DCs imprinted by transmissible ER stress are admixed with tumor cells and injected *in vivo*, facilitation of tumor growth is observed. Thus, tumor-borne ER stress plays a hitherto unappreciated role at the tumor/immune interface that ultimately facilitates tumor growth.

Keywords: ER stress; unfolded protein response; myeloid cells; dendritic cells; cross-priming; tumor growth facilitation; proinflammatory cytokines; arginase

Introduction

Eukaryotic cells react to endoplasmic reticulum (ER) stress by engaging a conserved set of intracellular signaling pathways known collectively as the unfolded protein response (UPR). ER stress response/UPR signaling pathways are activated in primary solid tumors as a result of cell-intrinsic defects, such as dysregulation of protein synthesis, folding and secretion, and aberrant glycosylation, but also microenvironmental noxae such as nutrient (e.g., glucose) deprivation, imbalance between demand and supply of oxygen (hypoxia), and imbalance between the production of reactive oxygen and the cell's ability to readily detoxify reactive intermediates (oxidative stress).[1] Some viruses that cause chronic infection also induce ER stress.[2]

In mammalian cells, the UPR is initiated by three ER membrane–bound sensors, IRE1α, ATF6, and PERK, which, in unstressed cells, are maintained in an inactive state through luminal association with the ER chaperone molecule GRP78.[3] When a cell experiences ER stress, GRP78 disassociates from each of the three sensor molecules to preferentially bind un/misfolded proteins, allowing each sensor to activate downstream signaling cascades, which act to normalize protein folding and secretion. PERK phosphorylates eIF2α, which results in selective inhibition of translation, effectively reducing ER client protein load. IRE1α autophosphorylates, activating its endonuclease to cleave Xbp-1 to generate a shortened Xbp-1 isoform (Xbp-1s), which drives the production of various ER chaperones to restore ER homeostasis. ATF6 translocates to the Golgi where it is cleaved into its functional form, which acts in parallel with Xbp-1s to restore ER homeostasis.[4] If ER stress persists, downstream signaling from PERK via ATF4 can also activate the transcription factor,

doi: 10.1111/nyas.12103

Ann. N.Y. Acad. Sci. 1284 (2013) 6–11 © 2013 New York Academy of Sciences.

Table 1. Links between the UPR and mechanisms of tumorigenesis

Cell-intrinsic events	Cell-extrinsic events
Adaptation of cellular energetics	Tumor promoting inflammation
Genomic instability and mutation	Evasion of antitumor immunity
Insensitivity to antigrowth signals	Promotion of angiogenesis
Self-sufficiency in growth signals	
Replicative immortality (telomerase activation)	
Evasion of apoptosis	
Tissue invasion and metastasis	

C/EBP homologous protein (CHOP), which can initiate apoptosis. Thus, if ER stress is too intense or protracted, compensatory mechanisms fail and cells undergo apoptosis.[3]

Substantial evidence implicates the UPR in tumorigenesis and cancer progression.[5] Breast cancers, possibly as a consequence of hypoxia, possess high levels of GRP78;[6] and proliferating and dormant cancer cells in which GRP78 is upregulated are resistant to chemotherapy.[7] The conditional homozygous knockout of *Grp78* in the prostate of mice with *Pten* inactivation protects against cancer growth,[8] whereas the inactivation, or a dominant-negative form, of PERK in cancer cells yields smaller and less aggressive tumors in mice.[9] Moreover, the inactivation of PERK and IRE1α results in impaired tumor cell survival under hypoxic conditions *in vitro* and decreased tumor growth *in vivo*.[9,10] The links between the UPR and tumorigenesis, cancer growth, and progression can be divided into two major categories. In the first category are the cell-intrinsic effects that include the more canonical links between the UPR and cancer, which are recognized to promote direct survival advantages (Table 1). The second category relates to the emerging role of the UPR in orchestrating inflammation in the tumor microenvironment, promoting evasion of antitumor immunity, and sustaining angiogenesis

(Table 1). These cell-extrinsic effects are less clearly understood.

Although evidence that the UPR may regulate immunity is still limited,[11] effects of the UPR on antigen presenting cells[12] and T cells[13,14] have been reported. Since both innate and adaptive immune responses play a crucial role in antitumor defense, and their subversion leads to tumor escape, it is important to define the role of the UPR in the context of antitumor immunity. This review will briefly recapitulate work from our laboratory, specifically highlighting the relation between the tumor UPR and immune cells, with emphasis on myeloid (CD11b$^+$) and CD8 T cells. These studies initially focused on myeloid cells, owing to the fact that these cells, including macrophages and dendritic cells (DCs), infiltrate solid tumors, and under the influence of tumor-derived signals, polarize to a phenotype that facilitates tumor growth.[15] In this context, tumor-infiltrating DCs inhibit T cell proliferation even though the signals necessary for efficient T cell priming are apparently in place.[16,17] The work discussed here suggests that tumor-borne UPR is a new determinant of the tumor/immune interface, serving as a new interpretative tool for the phenomenology of the tumor microenvironment as it relates to tumor growth and progression.

A cell-extrinsic effect of tumor UPR on myeloid cells

A previously unappreciated cell-extrinsic effect of the tumor UPR is its transmission to myeloid cells, such as macrophages and DCs.[18,19] This new phenomenon, transmissible ER stress (TERS), was discovered while investigating the effects of conditioned medium from ER stressed murine tumor cells (e.g., prostate, melanoma, lung carcinoma) on bone marrow–derived macrophages and DCs. Cancer cells were stressed using thapsigargin, a sesquiterpene lactone canonical ER stress inducer that inhibits the sarco/endoplasmic reticulum Ca^{2+} ATPase, and glucose starvation. We found that bone marrow–derived macrophages and DCs both function as receivers of TERS to which they respond by mounting a global ER stress response, characterized by transcriptional upregulation of the master UPR regulator Grp78 and two downstream UPR effectors, Xbp-1s and CHOP. Cancer cells under ER stress also upregulate a proinflammatory gene program, including the protumorigenic cytokines

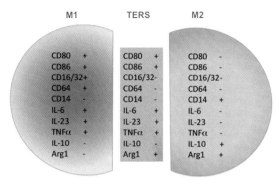

Figure 1. Phenotypic characteristics of TERS-imprinted, bone marrow–derived macrophages, and comparison with the canonical characteristics of M1 and M2 macrophages. Data shown with permission from Mahadevan *et al.*[18]

IL-6, IL-23p19, and TNF-α.[20] Other cytokines/chemokines, such as TGF-β, MIP-1α, MIP-1β and MCP-1, are also increased, while there is no effect on IL-10. Importantly, TERS also caused the upregulation of arginase I in both macrophages and DCs.[18, 19] Since arginase I is a suppressor of T cell function,[21] we concluded that TERS imparts myeloid cells with a proinflammatory/suppressive phenotype.[22]

TERS-imprinted, bone marrow–derived DCs rapidly change morphology, acquiring characteristics of activated, mature DCs, including increased cell size and elongated dendrites.[18] They also upregulate expression of major histocompatibility complex (MHC) classes I and II, and the costimulatory molecules CD86, CD80, and, to a lesser extent, CD40. These cells are CD8α−, confirming their myeloid origin. The general phenotypic features of CD11b+ cells, macrophages, and DCs upon TERS imprinting are summarized in Figure 1. TERS-imprinted myeloid cells do not upregulate GR-1, distinguishing their phenotype from that of classical myeloid-derived suppressor cells (MDSC).[23] PD-L1, the ligand for the T cell immunoinhibitory PD-1 receptor,[24] is only slightly increased in TERS-imprinted, bone marrow–derived DCs.[18]

TERS imprinting affects antigen presentation by DCs

Experiments performed on bone marrow–derived DCs led to the unanticipated finding that TERS-imprinting adversely affects cross-presentation and cross-priming.[18] Cross-presentation was studied in a system in which the ovalbumin (OVA) SIINFEKL peptide, bound to the H2-K^b molecule, can be detected by the monoclonal antibody 25-D1.16. Reproducibly, we found reduced display of the SIINFEKL/H2-K^b complex at the cell surface of OVA-fed, TERS-imprinted, bone marrow–derived DCs, while the expression of MHC class I molecules remained constant or even increased over that of OVA-fed control DCs.[18] Using the OVA system and CD8+ T cells from OT-I mice whose T cell receptor (TCR) is specific for the SIINFEKL/H2-K^b complex, we investigated the ability of TERS-imprinting to affect CD8+ T cell cross-priming by bone marrow–derived DCs *in vitro* (Fig. 2, upper panel).[18] As expected, OVA-fed, bone marrow–derived DCs, unstimulated or treated with the conditioned medium of unstressed tumor cells, efficiently induced both activation and proliferation of OT-I T cells, as determined by surface staining for CD69, CD25, CD62L and CD44, and by 5-(and-6)-carboxyfluorescein diacetate, succinimidyl ester (CFDA-SE) dilution.[18] In contrast, OT-I T cells cocultured with OVA-fed, TERS-imprinted, bone marrow–derived DCs proliferated poorly while activated, resulting in a higher (>70%) percentage of activated, nondividing T cells.[18] PD-1 was not upregulated in T cells. The proliferation defect could be restored by adding exogenous antigen (1 mg/mL), but not by adding exogenous IL-2 during cross-priming, arguing against classical T cell anergy.[25] The proliferation defect was further rescued (∼80%) by L-norvaline, a competitive inhibitor of arginase I, but surprisingly, not by the addition of L-arginine.[18] Thus, tumor-borne UPR is transmitted to myeloid cells, which, in turn, produce arginase I, contributing to the T cell proliferation defect observed (Fig. 2, lower panel).

Initial studies on fate determination of CD8 T cells cross-primed by TERS-imprinted DCs

Using the *in vitro* system described previously, we determined that T cells cross-primed by TERS-imprinted, bone marrow–derived DCs upregulate transcription of various cytokines, including IL-10 and TNF-α, but not IL-17. They also upregulate Foxp3 while downregulating CD28. LAG3, a negative regulator of TCR signaling on tumor-infiltrating CD8+ T cells,[26] was only slightly upregulated. A provisional conclusion is that CD8 T cells cross-primed by TERS-imprinted, bone marrow–derived DCs display an uncommitted phenotype with potential suppressive characteristics

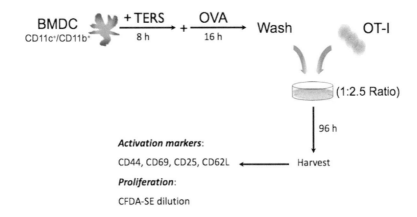

	Control DC	TERS DC
CD69	+++	+++
CD44	+++	+++
CD25	+++	+++
CD62L	±	+
CFDA-SE dilution	+++	+
PD-1	--	--
LAG3	--	--

Figure 2. Characteristics of CD8[+] T cells cross-primed *in vitro* by TERS-imprinted, bone marrow–derived DCs (BMDCs). Upper panel: diagram illustrating the experimental procedure for cross-priming of OT-I CD8[+] T cells using TERS-imprinted DCs. Lower panel: phenotypic and proliferative characteristics of CD8[+] T cells cross-primed *in vitro* by TERS-imprinted DCs. Control DCs comprise both DCs that received no treatment (regular cross-priming) and DCs treated with vehicle-conditioned medium. (–) = no appreaciable variation from controls. Data shown with permission from Mahadevan *et al.*[18]

(CD28 downregulation and IL-10 upregulation), which render them similar to CD8[+]/CD28[−] regulatory T cells secreting IL-10 and TNF-α, and expressing FOXP3 that have been found to infiltrate a variety of human tumors.[27,28]

Tumor growth facilitation

In a direct test of whether immune cells facilitate tumor growth *in vivo*,[29] we subcutaneously inoculated C57/BL6 mice with B16.F10 tumor cells admixed with TERS-imprinted, bone marrow–derived DCs; not surprisingly, this resulted in faster tumor growth, earlier tumor initiation, and decreased survival of mice.[18] Furthermore, the inoculation of mice with TC1.OVA prostate cancer cells, constitutively expressing the OVA rejection antigen, caused transient tumor growth only when admixed with TERS-imprinted, bone marrow–derived DCs.[18] This suggests that one of the effects of TERS is to induce dysfunctional CD8[+] T cells, which ultimately may provide for immune escape by the tumor cells.

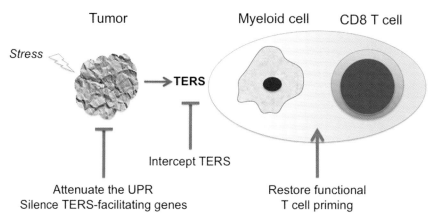

Figure 3. Diagram illustrating the potential benefits of therapeutic interventions directed at the tumor UPR and its cell-extrinsic effects such as TERS.

Conclusions

Recent work from our laboratory points to a role for the tumor UPR on myeloid cells and CD8+ T cells. The ensemble of these effects stems from the cell-extrinsic effects of the tumor UPR, and represents a new way through which tumor cells, under the umbrella of the UPR, can affect both myeloid cells and CD8+ T cells.[22] Paradoxically, the defect of bone marrow–derived DCs deriving from TERS imprinting differ from that of tolerogenic DCs, which have been described as steady-state immature cells able to present antigen.[30] In contrast, TERS-imprinted, bone marrow–derived DCs are phenotypically mature cells with diminished capacity of cross-presenting antigen and cross-priming CD8+ T cells. Thus, cell-extrinsic signals borne out of tumor UPR can recapitulate *ab initio* the activated/suppressive phenotype observed in tumor-infiltrating myeloid cells *in vivo*.[16] The extent to which TERS-mediated functional incapacitation of myeloid cells induces immune evasion is not known at this time and will require further work. However, because the tumor UPR induces, through TERS, several of the immune defects observed in the tumor microenvironment,[22] new attention must be directed at therapies that target the UPR to effectively curb tumor cells adaptation and survival *in vivo*[31] and to control immune suppression due to the cell extrinsic effects of the tumor UPR (Fig. 3). It is not difficult to imagine that this new type of control of the tumor microenvironment will effectively aid the generation and persistence of spontaneous, or vaccine-induced, antitumor T cell responses.

Acknowledgment

I am particularly grateful to Dr. Navin R. Mahadevan for his dedicated work and insights into the new field of medical exploration reflected in the synthesis presented at the 2012 Cancer Vaccine Symposium. I thank Jeffrey J. Rodvold, Veronika Anufreichik, and Homero Sepulveda for their contributions to the performance of the experiments. This work was supported by a grant from the UCSD Academic Senate.

Conflicts of interest

The author declares no conflicts of interest.

References

1. Heazlewood, C.K., M.C. Cook, R. Eri, *et al.* 2008. Aberrant mucin assembly in mice causes endoplasmic reticulum stress and spontaneous inflammation resembling ulcerative colitis. *PLoS Med.* **5:** e54.
2. He, B. 2006. Viruses, endoplasmic reticulum stress, and interferon responses. *Cell Death Differ.* **13:** 393–403.
3. Walter, P. & D. Ron. 2011. The unfolded protein response: from stress pathway to homeostatic regulation. *Science* **334:** 1081–1086.
4. Yamamoto, K., T. Sato, T. Matsui, *et al.* 2007. Transcriptional induction of mammalian ER quality control proteins is mediated by single or combined action of ATF6alpha and XBP1. *Dev. Cell* **13:** 365–376.
5. Germain, R.N., E.A. Robey & M.D. Cahalan. 2012. A decade of imaging cellular motility and interaction dynamics in the immune system. *Science* **336:** 1676–1681.
6. Li, J. & A. S. Lee. 2006. Stress induction of GRP78/BiP and its role in cancer. *Curr. Mol. Med.* **6:** 45–54.
7. Ranganathan, A.C., L. Zhang, A.P. Adam, & J.A. Aguirre-Ghiso. 2006. Functional coupling of p38-induced upregulation of BiP and activation of RNA-dependent protein

kinase-like endoplasmic reticulum kinase to drug resistance of dormant carcinoma cells. *Cancer Res.* **66:** 1702–1711.

8. Fu, Y., S. Wey, M. Wang, *et al.* 2008. Pten null prostate tumorigenesis and AKT activation are blocked by targeted knockout of ER chaperone GRP78/BiP in prostate epithelium. *Proc. Natl. Acad. Sci. USA* **105:** 19444–19449.

9. Bi, M., C. Naczki, M. Koritzinsky, *et al.* 2005. ER stress-regulated translation increases tolerance to extreme hypoxia and promotes tumor growth. *EMBO J.* **24:** 3470–3481.

10. Romero-Ramirez, L., H. Cao, D. Nelson, *et al.* 2004. XBP1 is essential for survival under hypoxic conditions and is required for tumor growth. *Cancer Res.* **64:** 5943–5947.

11. Todd, D.J., A.H. Lee & L.H. Glimcher 2008. The endoplasmic reticulum stress response in immunity and autoimmunity. *Nat. Rev. Immunol.* **8:** 663–674.

12. Wheeler, M.C., M. Rizzi, R. Sasik, *et al.* 2008. KDEL-retained antigen in B lymphocytes induces a proinflammatory response: a possible role for endoplasmic reticulum stress in adaptive T cell immunity. *J. Immunol.* **181:** 256–264.

13. Kamimura, D. & M.J. Bevan 2008. Endoplasmic reticulum stress regulator XBP-1 contributes to effector CD8[+] T cell differentiation during acute infection. *J. Immunol.* **181:** 5433–5441.

14. Franco, A., G. Almanza, J.C. Burns, *et al.* 2010. Endoplasmic reticulum stress drives a regulatory phenotype in human T-cell clones. *Cell Immunol.* **266:** 1–6.

15. Ostrand-Rosenberg, S. & P. Sinha. 2009. Myeloid-derived suppressor cells: linking inflammation and cancer. *J. Immunol.* **182:** 4499–4506.

16. Norian, L.A., P.C. Rodriguez, L.A. O'Mara, *et al.* 2009. Tumor-infiltrating regulatory dendritic cells inhibit CD8[+] T cell function via L-arginine metabolism. *Cancer Res.* **69:** 3086–3094.

17. Liu, Q., C. Zhang, A. Sun, *et al.* 2009. Tumor-educated CD11bhighIalow regulatory dendritic cells suppress T cell response through arginase I. *J. Immunol.* **182:** 6207–6216.

18. Mahadevan, N.R., V. Anufreichik, J.J. Rodvold, *et al.* 2012. Cell extrinsic effect of tumor ER stress imprint myeloid dendritic cells and impair CD8 T cell priming. *PLoS One* **7:** e51845.

19. Mahadevan, N.R., J. Rodvold, H. Sepulveda, *et al.* 2011. Transmission of endoplasmic reticulum stress and pro-inflammation from tumor cells to myeloid cells. *Proc. Natl. Acad. Sci. USA* **108:** 6561–6566.

20. Mahadevan, N.R., A. Fernandez, J. Rodvold, *et al.* 2010. Prostate cells undergoing ER stress in vitro and in vivo activate transcription of pro-inflammatory cytokines. *J. Inflam. Res.* **3:** 99–103.

21. Bronte, V. & P. Zanovello. 2005. Regulation of immune responses by L-arginine metabolism. *Nat. Rev. Immunol.* **5:** 641–654.

22. Mahadevan, N.R. & M. Zanetti. 2011. Tumor stress inside out: cell-extrinsic effects of the unfolded protein response in tumor cells modulate the immunological landscape of the tumor microenvironment. *J. Immunol.* **187:** 4403–4409.

23. Gabrilovich, D.I., S. Ostrand-Rosenberg & V. Bronte. 2012. Coordinated regulation of myeloid cells by tumours. *Nat. Rev. Immunol.* **12:** 253–268.

24. Freeman, G.J., A.J. Long, Y. Iwai, *et al.* 2000. Engagement of the PD-1 immunoinhibitory receptor by a novel B7 family member leads to negative regulation of lymphocyte activation. *J. Exp. Med.* **192:** 1027–1034.

25. Beverly, B., S.M. Kang, M.J. Lenardo & R.H. Schwartz. 1992. Reversal of in vitro T cell clonal anergy by IL-2 stimulation. *Int. Immunol.* **4:** 661–671.

26. Grosso, J.F., C.C. Kelleher, T.J. Harris, *et al.* 2007. LAG-3 regulates CD8[+] T cell accumulation and effector function in murine self- and tumor-tolerance systems. *J. Clin. Invest.* **117:** 3383–3392.

27. Filaci, G., D. Fenoglio, M. Fravega, *et al.* 2007. CD8[+] CD28- T regulatory lymphocytes inhibiting T cell proliferative and cytotoxic functions infiltrate human cancers. *J. Immunol.* **179:** 4323–4334.

28. Mahic, M., K. Henjum, S. Yaqub, *et al.* 2008. Generation of highly suppressive adaptive CD8(+)CD25(+)FOXP3(+) regulatory T cells by continuous antigen stimulation. *Eur. J. Immunol.* **38:** 640–646.

29. Prehn, R.T. 1972. The immune reaction as a stimulator of tumor growth. *Science* **176:** 170–171.

30. Steinman, R.M. & M.C. Nussenzweig. 2002. Avoiding horror autotoxicus: the importance of dendritic cells in peripheral T cell tolerance. *Proc. Natl. Acad. Sci. USA* **99:** 351–358.

31. Healy, S.J., A.M. Gorman, P. Mousavi-Shafaei, *et al.* 2009. Targeting the endoplasmic reticulum-stress response as an anticancer strategy. *Eur. J. Pharmacol.* **625:** 234–246.

Ann. N.Y. Acad. Sci. ISSN 0077-8923

ANNALS OF THE NEW YORK ACADEMY OF SCIENCES

Issue: *The Renaissance of Cancer Immunotherapy*

Immunotherapy in preneoplastic disease: targeting early procarcinogenic inflammatory changes that lead to immune suppression and tumor tolerance

Bridget Keenan[1,2,3] and Elizabeth M. Jaffee[1,2,4]

[1]The Sidney Kimmel Cancer Center at Johns Hopkins, [2]Department of Oncology, [3]Graduate Program in Immunology, and [4]The Skip Viragh Pancreatic Cancer Center, Johns Hopkins University School of Medicine, Baltimore, Maryland

Address for correspondence: Elizabeth M. Jaffee, M.D., Department of Oncology, Johns Hopkins University School of Medicine, The Sidney Kimmel Cancer Center at Johns Hopkins, 4M07 Bunting Blaustein Cancer Research Building, 1650 Orleans St., Baltimore, MD 21287. ejaffee@jhmi.edu

Recent advances in immunotherapy have demonstrated that single agent vaccines can be effective when given as primary prevention before exposure to the causative agent, and partially effective in some patients with existing cancer. However, as tumors develop and progress, tumor-induced immune suppression and tolerance present the greatest barrier to therapeutic success. Preneoplastic disease represents an important opportunity to intervene with tumor antigen–targeted vaccines before these mechanisms of immune evasion outpace efforts by the immune system to destroy precancerous cells. However, as we discuss in this review, emerging evidence suggests that procarcinogenic inflammatory changes occur early in cancer development, in both patients and mouse models of cancer progression. Defining early inhibitory signals within tumor microenvironments will yield insights that can eventually be used in the clinic to target these events and deliver treatments that can be used in addition to cancer vaccines to prevent premalignant and early invasive cancers.

Keywords: cancer vaccines; preneoplasia; immunotherapy; pancreatic cancer

Introduction

The recent FDA-approval of two immunotherapies for cancer treatment has established immunotherapy as a legitimate therapeutic modality as well as an emerging and exciting area of clinical research with a rich pipeline that may yield many new cancer drugs. Yet, despite this progress, immune-based therapies so far have demonstrated only limited success in the clinic. One reason for this failure is that clinical trials testing immune-based therapies typically study patient populations with advanced disease who have failed many prior therapies, indicating that their cancer is already resistant to multiple treatment modalities. A second explanation is based on the recent discovery that mechanisms of immune evasion and suppression develop earlier than previously thought, at the time of the earliest stages of cancer development. These findings from preclinical models and advanced cancer patients imply that multiple mechanisms of immune tolerance have been established by the time of cancer diagnosis. With improved screening techniques and the discovery of new biomarkers and genetic signatures defining different cancer biologies, there is hope for detection and treatment of cancer in its premalignant or early invasive stages. Immunotherapy aimed at this population should be based on knowledge of early suppressive signaling events present in preneoplasia; thus, continued investigation into these early networks may be essential for successful development of early immunologic interventions.

Lessons learned from virally associated cancers

Cancer vaccines are inherently different than vaccines for infectious disease. Most vaccines for

doi: 10.1111/nyas.12076

Ann. N.Y. Acad. Sci. 1284 (2013) 12–16 © 2013 New York Academy of Sciences.

infectious disease are used in a primary prevention setting and given in childhood before disease exposure. They induce neutralizing antibody responses to clear infections before they can cause harm. However, much can be learned from the use of immunotherapy to treat persistent viral infections and the cancers that can arise as a result. Vaccines for established or chronic infection have a much lower success rate than those administered for primary prevention, as with the example of human papilloma virus (HPV) vaccination. The two FDA-approved vaccines for HPV are aimed at young adolescents with the goal of decreasing sexually transmitted disease and ultimately, HPV-associated cancers. In populations with no exposure to the HPV strains targeted by the vaccine, there is greater than 90% efficacy for prevention of infection and cervical intraepithelial neoplasia (CIN).[1] However, in studies of all women who were vaccinated regardless of HPV infection status, this rate dropped to 50% or lower, due to ineffectiveness in previously or currently infected individuals.[1] Although this has likely contributed to the design of the preventive HPV vaccine, which elicits neutralizing antibodies, other HPV vaccines attempting to enhance the cellular immune response as therapeutic interventions have had similarly low rates of success. In one trial administering a DNA vaccine targeting mutated E7 to women with HPV16$^+$ CIN stage two and three (CIN2/3), the rates of regression following vaccination with the highest dose were 33%, slightly higher than the rate of spontaneous regression in historical controls (25%).[2]

Foreign antigens are more likely to elicit a powerful immune response than self-antigens from spontaneously occurring cancers, making virally related cancers an ideal candidate for the use of cancer vaccines. However, even early on in persistent infections, before the development of cancer, there is downregulation of CD8$^+$ T cell responses to viral antigens, resulting in viral immune escape. Hepatitis C infection often becomes chronic, leading to liver fibrosis, and eventually in some cases, hepatocellular carcinoma. The standard of treatment for hepatitis C infection has been, for many years, pegylated interferon-alpha, a potent immunostimulator, and ribavirin, an antiviral; this combination results in viral clearance and recovery in 43–80% of infected individuals, depending on viral genotype.[3] As in other persistent infections such as HIV, T cells in hepatitis C–infected patients demonstrate markers of exhaustion and decreased activation, such as impaired cytokine secretion and upregulated immune checkpoint markers, including PD-1, CTLA-4, and TIM-3.[3] Despite the role of the immune system in eliminating these viral infections and preventing virally associated cancers, there are early events that prevent the maximum function of the immune response, creating barriers to treatment by immunotherapy.

Targeting early oncogene expression in cancer development

With the advent of technically superior sequencing techniques, there has been rapid progress in the characterization of genetic mutations in many tumor types. This provides a framework of initiating genetic alterations, including oncogene activation or tumor suppressor loss, which can be targeted with immunotherapy earlier in disease. Interventions made within this window of opportunity could prevent preneoplastic lesions from progressing to cancer, a strategy that could be particularly useful for populations known to be at increased risk for particular types of cancer. However, results from the few attempts at vaccination against precancer, both in preclinical models and clinical trials, have overall been ineffective, but also provide valuable insights into how these vaccination strategies can be improved.

In addition to clinical trials for CIN2/3, a precursor to cervical cancer, cancer vaccines have been used in a clinical setting for ductal carcinoma *in situ* (DCIS), a noninvasive breast cancer that has the potential to become invasive. In a trial of a dendritic cell vaccine targeting HER-2/*neu*, 18.5% of patients had a complete response following vaccination, with lower rates in patients who had estrogen receptor–positive DCIS.[4] HER-2/*neu* expression was downregulated in 50% of patients who had residual DCIS, suggesting vaccination could induce immunoediting in cancers that were not eradicated by the immune system.[4] In preclinical treatment models, there have been similar findings on the partial efficacy of cancer vaccines in the course of cancer progression. In a mouse model of spontaneous colon cancer, intervention with a dendritic cell vaccine prevented progression to colon cancer by reducing the total number of intestinal polyps.[5] However, the vaccine, which targets an overexpressed protein in

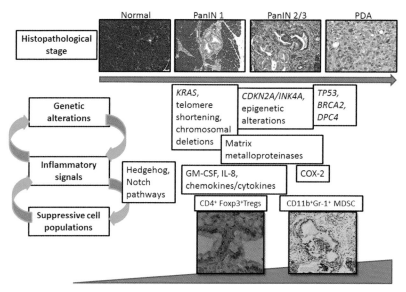

Figure 1. Inflammatory progression model for pancreatic ductal adenocarcinoma (PDA). Previous models have described the timing of genetic alterations in relation to different PanIN stages, which represent increasing degrees of cellular atypia, loss of normal tissue structure, and genetic abnormality. We propose a new model incorporating the relationship between genetic mutations and gene expression changes with inflammatory cytokines and signaling present in the tumor microenvironment, as well as with cell populations recruited to the tumor microenvironment. Using PDA as an example, we show that genetic mutations, such as *Kras*, can induce secretion of inflammatory cytokines, such as GM-CSF and IL-8, which induce and recruit immature myeloid and granulocytic cells, as well as suppressive T$_{reg}$ cells, that then drive immune tolerance and escape. These procarcinogenic immune cells can contribute to an inflammatory milieu, that is capable of suppressing effector T cell responses, recruiting additional suppressive cells, modifying tumor vasculature, and contributing to further DNA damage and mutations, all of which results in cancer progression.

colon cancer and induced CD4$^+$ and CD8$^+$ T cell responses, did not result in a statistically significant increase in survival.[5] Thus, there is increasing evidence that mechanisms of treatment resistance and immune evasion that occur in advanced cancers are also present to some degree in preoplastic conditions. As the use of immunotherapy in preneoplasia moves forward, it will become increasingly important to define what these suppressive signals are and identify druggable targets for use in combination with vaccination.

Barriers to prevention of cancer progression by cancer vaccines

Pancreatic ductal adenocarcinoma (PDA) is characterized by an intense desmoplastic response that occurs in the stroma, presenting unique challenges for drug delivery and effective treatment. Mouse models of spontaneous developing pancreatic cancer have been genetically engineered and are based on expression of dominant active K-Ras and loss of p53 expression, two common genetic alterations in human PDA.[6,7] These mouse models recapitulate

the progression to PDA via pancreatic intraepithelial neoplasia (PanIN) stages one, two, and three, accompanied by increasing genetic and cellular abnormalities, as well as the characteristic stromal reaction.[7] This model, therefore, provides an opportunity to define the sequential events that contribute to a suppressive tumor microenvironment, which is poorly vascularized and highly treatment resistant. As observed in many other cancers, CD4$^+$Foxp3$^+$ T regulatory (T$_{reg}$) cells and CD11b$^+$Gr-1$^+$ cells are two dominant populations infiltrating cancers, but they are also present in PanINs.[7] Studies in this mouse model of PDA have revealed that granulocyte macrophage colony-stimulating factor (GM-CSF) is secreted by tumors, which in turn, recruits CD11b$^+$Gr-1$^+$ cells responsible for impairing CD8$^+$ T cell function and barring their infiltration into tumors.[8]

In addition, the PDA mouse model recapitulates the early expression of the *Kras^{G12D}* oncogene mutation, known to occur early in human PDA development. Mutated *Kras* is present in approximately 40% of early stage, and 87% of late stage, PanINs in humans, and likely contributes to GM-CSF secretion, early infiltration of the CD11b$^+$Gr-1$^+$ cells, and T cell suppression.[6] K-Ras has also been shown to induce production of IL-8, a transcriptional target of this oncogene,[9] and a known attractant of granulocytes and macrophages, providing another mechanism for recruiting suppressive immune cells to the developing tumor.[9] Work is ongoing in our laboratory and others to more completely characterize these cells infiltrating the site of pancreatic tumor development and the signals that recruit them to PanINs, so as to build on genetic and histopathological models of cancer progression with an additional inflammatory progression model (Fig. 1).

In addition to recruiting suppressive immune cell populations, developing tumors alter the microenvironment in other ways to evade the protective antitumor response. CIN2/3 patients who had spontaneous regression of their cervical lesions had weak T cell responses to E6 and E7 antigens in their blood, yet were found to harbor extensive CD8$^+$ T cell infiltrates in cervical epithelium.[10] Lesions that persisted were characterized by the absence of CD8$^+$ T cells and downregulation of MAdCAM-1, the receptor for $\alpha_4\beta_7$ integrin, which is expressed by CD8$^+$ T cells infiltrating cervical tissue.[10] Thus, in these early lesions that do not regress, the dysplastic epithelium has already developed mechanisms for excluding CD8$^+$ T cells and evading the immune system.

Additional barriers to T cell activation, both systemically and within tumor microenvironment, include immune checkpoint molecules, such as CTLA-4, PD-1, and LAG-3, which dampen T cell signaling following antigen recognition. Tumors upregulate inhibitory ligands for these T cell checkpoint molecules, representing an adaptive strategy to inhibit T cell activation. With the U.S. Food and Drug Administration (FDA) approval of anti-CTLA-4 for metastatic melanoma and trials investigating drugs to target other immune checkpoints, monoclonal antibodies against immune checkpoints represent a novel class of cancer therapeutics. In the future, it is likely that we will see the combined use of cancer vaccines to stimulate an antitumor T cell response and the blockade of immune checkpoints to overcome inhibitory signaling encountered within the tumor microenvironment. As research continues in this field, we may find that immune checkpoints are also expressed in preneoplasia and warrant targeting in combination with vaccination, even in early disease.

Conclusions

Over the past few years, the opportunities for the use of immunotherapy in cancer have expanded. However, challenges to effective treatment remain in the form of suppressive tumor microenvironments, and infiltrating cell populations induced and recruited by tumor signaling. In addition, we are discovering that these suppressive signaling networks begin early in the progression of cancer. This window of time before cancer has progressed provides an ideal setting for the use of immunotherapy while there is a role for the protective antitumor immune response. Combination immunotherapy to induce potent CD8$^+$ T cell responses and to target suppressive signaling will be necessary, even at the earliest stages, to switch off the progression to cancer and immune evasion, and turn on mechanisms that eliminate preneoplasia. As the ability to detect and treat early stage cancers increases, interventions used in combination with traditional cancer therapies or vaccines should include agents that modulate the early suppressive events occurring in cancer development. Continuing to define what these signals are is critical for building a model of inflammatory progression.

Conflicts of interest

E.M.J. receives commercial consulting fees from Bristol-Meyers-Squibb (Pancreatic Advisory Board Consultant), has the potential to receive royalties, milestone payments, and travel reimbursement from BioSante and Aduro Biotech (compliance governed by Johns Hopkins University Conflict of Interest Committee).

References

1. Tsu, V., M. Murray & S. Franceschi. 2012. Human papillomavirus vaccination in low-resource countries: lack of evidence to support vaccinating sexually active women. *Br. J. Cancer.* **107:** 1445–1450.

2. Trimble, C.L., S. Peng, F. Kos, *et al.* 2009. A phase I trial of a human papillomavirus DNA vaccine for HPV16$^+$ cervical intraepithelial neoplasia 2/3. *Clin. Cancer Res.* **15:** 361–367.

3. Ip, P.P., H.W. Nijman, J. Wilschut, *et al.* 2012. Therapeutic vaccination against chronic hepatitis C virus infection. *Antiviral Res.* **96:** 36–50.

4. Sharma, A., U. Koldovsky, S. Xu, *et al.* 2012. HER-2 pulsed dendritic cell vaccine can eliminate HER-2 expression and impact ductal carcinoma in situ. *Cancer* **118:** 4354–4362.

5. Yokomine, K., T. Nakatsura, S. Senju, *et al.* 2007. Regression of intestinal adenomas by vaccination with heat shock protein 105-pulsed bone marrow-derived dendritic cells in Apc(Min/+) mice. *Cancer Sci.* **98:** 1930–1935.

6. Feldmann, G., R. Beaty, R.H. Hruban, *et al.* 2007. Molecular genetics of pancreatic intraepithelial neoplasia. *J. Hepatobiliary Pancreat. Surg.* **14:** 224–232.

7. Clark, C.E., S.R. Hingorani, R. Mick, *et al.* 2007. Dynamics of the immune reaction to pancreatic cancer from inception to invasion. *Cancer Res.* **67:** 9518–9527.

8. Bayne, L.J., G.L. Beatty, N. Jhala, *et al.* 2012. Tumor-derived granulocyte-macrophage colony-stimulating factor regulates myeloid inflammation and T cell immunity in pancreatic cancer. *Cancer Cell* **21:** 822–835.

9. Sparmann, A. & D. Bar-Sagi. 2004. Ras-induced interleukin-8 expression plays a critical role in tumor growth and angiogenesis. *Cancer Cell* **6:** 447–458.

10. Trimble, C.L., R.A. Clark, C. Thoburn, *et al.* 2010. Human papillomavirus 16-associated cervical intraepithelial neoplasia in humans excludes CD8 T cells from dysplastic epithelium. *J. Immunol.* **185:** 7107–7114.

Ann. N.Y. Acad. Sci. ISSN 0077-8923

Integration of epidemiology, immunobiology, and translational research for brain tumors

Hideho Okada,[1] Michael E. Scheurer,[2] Saumendra N. Sarkar,[1] and Melissa L. Bondy[2]

[1]University of Pittsburgh Cancer Institute, Pittsburgh, Pennsylvania. [2]Dan L. Duncan Cancer Center at Baylor College of Medicine, Houston, Texas

Address for correspondence: Hideho Okada, University of Pittsburgh School of Medicine, Hillman Cancer Center, 5117 Centre Avenue, Pittsburgh, PA 15213. okadah@upmc.edu

We recently identified a pivotal role for the host type I interferon (IFN) pathway in immunosurveillance against *de novo* mouse glioma development, especially through the regulation of immature myeloid cells (IMCs) in the glioma microenvironment. The present paper summarizes our published work in a number of areas. We have identified single-nucleotide polymorphisms (SNPs) in human IFN genes that dictate altered prognosis of patients with glioma. One of these SNPs (rs12553612) is located in the promoter of *IFNA8* and influences its activity. Conversely, recent epidemiologic data show that chronic use of nonsteroidal anti-inflammatory drugs lowers the risk of glioma. We translated these findings back to our *de novo* glioma model and found that cyclooxygenase-2 inhibition enhances antiglioma immunosurveillance by reducing glioma-associated IMCs. Taken together, these findings suggest that alterations in myeloid cell function condition the brain for glioma development. Finally, in preliminary work, we have begun applying novel immunotherapeutic approaches to patients with low-grade glioma with the aim of preventing malignant transformation. Future research will hopefully better integrate epidemiological, immunobiological, and translational techniques to develop novel, preventive approaches for malignant gliomas.

Keywords: interferon; glioma; nonsteroidal antiinflammatory drugs; single-nucleotide polymorphism

Inflammation-related genetic and immunologic factors in glioma development

Glioma accounts for approximately 40% of all primary brain tumors and are responsible for roughly 13,000 cancer-related deaths in the United States each year.[1] World Health Organization (WHO) grade IV glioblastoma (GBM) is the most common and most malignant of the glial tumors, with a median survival of 15 months. Other common types of malignant glioma are WHO grade III anaplastic glioma, including anaplastic astrocytoma, which has a median survival of 24–36 months. WHO grade II low-grade gliomas (LGGs) are slow-growing primary brain tumors with infiltrative growth characteristics in the brain, and therefore have an extremely high risk of progression following treatment with surgery, or surgery followed by radiation therapy (RT).[2–10] There is no curative treatment because these tumors grow invasively in the central nervous system (CNS). More than 50% of these patients eventually recur with aggressive WHO grade III or IV high-grade gliomas (HGGs),[6,7,11,12] and most LGG patients eventually die of the disease.

Predicting which populations are at risk for glioma is difficult: established risk factors (exposure to ionizing radiation, rare mutations of penetrant genes, and family history) account for only a small proportion of brain tumors.[13] Recent reports suggest the involvement of inflammation-related genetic and immunologic factors in gliomagenesis,[14–26] including studies by our group.[18,27–32] Interestingly, independent studies by multiple groups have reported similar observations as summarized below: (1) A history of asthma and allergies as well as higher immunoglobulin E levels have been inversely associated with glioma development and prognosis.[18,19,21,22,24,25] SNPs that

doi: 10.1111/nyas.12115

increase asthma risk also seem to be associated with reduced risk of glioma.[16] Downregulation of the majority of allergy- and inflammation-related genes is associated with more aggressive GBM progression.[14] Among populations reporting a history of asthma or allergies with asthma, regular long-term use of antihistamines is significantly associated with an increased risk for glioma;[28,29] (2) SNPs in interleukin-4 receptor-α (IL-4Rα) are associated with altered glioma risk and prognosis;[15,27] and (3) chronic use of nonsteroidal anti-inflammatory drugs (NSAIDs) is associated with reduced glioma risk.[17,28,29] Although these data point to a role for immunologic and genetic factors in gliomagenesis, the relationships among these factors, and the biological mechanisms underlying these observations, warrant further study.

Integration of mechanistic and epidemiological studies

Our goal is to fill an important gap in our mechanistic understanding of factors that influence the risk and prognosis of glioma identified through epidemiologic studies, and to translate these findings to the clinic through preclinical mouse and genomic studies as well as early phase clinical trials. To this end, we are working to integrate state-of-the-art human epidemiology, cell biology, and novel mouse glioma models in a thematic, hypothesis-driven manner.

Type I IFNs in immunological responses against glioma: preclinical mouse studies

We have long been interested in the role of type I interferons (IFNs) in immunological responses against glioma.[33–36] Using a novel *de novo* mouse glioma model,[37] we investigated the role of the type I IFN pathway in glioma development by inducing *de novo* gliomas in IFN-α receptor 1–deficient (*Ifnar1*[−/−]) mice. This study identified a pivotal role for the host IFN-α pathway in protecting against glioma development (Fig. 1A), especially through the downregulation of immature myeloid cells (IMCs; Fig. 1B), which most likely include myeloid-derived suppressor cells (MDSCs), in the glioma microenvironment.[30] Based on these data, we evaluated and identified SNPs in human *IFNA* genes associated with the prognosis of patients with glioma.[30] One of these SNPs, rs12553612, is located in the *IFNA8* promoter and is associated with better overall survival of glioma patients with the AA-genotype compared with patients with the AC-genotype (Fig. 1C).

We subsequently hypothesized that the A-allele allows for enhanced *IFNA8* promoter activity compared with the C-allele. We performed reporter assays in the human monocyte-derived THP-1

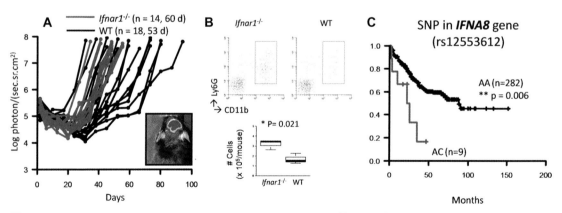

Figure 1. Effects of IFN-α gene alterations on glioma development in mice and humans. (A, B) Gliomas were induced in C57BL/6 background *Ifnar1*[−/−] (red lines) or wild-type (WT; black lines) neonatal mice by intraventricular transfection of plasmids: *pT2/C-Luc//PGK-SB1.a3* (0.2 µg), *pT/CAG-NRas* (0.4 µg), and *pT/shp53* (0.4 µg). (A) Tumor growth was monitored. (B) The mice bearing *SB*-induced tumors were sacrificed at days 50–60, and brain infiltrating leukocytes (BILs) were isolated based on similar tumor size observed by bioluminescence imaging (BLI). BILs obtained from three mice in a given group were pooled and evaluated by flow cytometry for CD11b[+]Ly6G[+] IMCs. Absolute IMC numbers in three independent experiments are depicted in the bottom panels. *P* values were based on Student's *t*-test. (C) Overall survival was evaluated among 291 glioma patients with WHO grade II–III gliomas by genotype for SNPs in *IFNA8* rs12553612. Patients with AC genotype (red line) exhibited a significantly shorter survival than those with the AA genotype (black line). Reproduced, with permission, from Ref. 30.

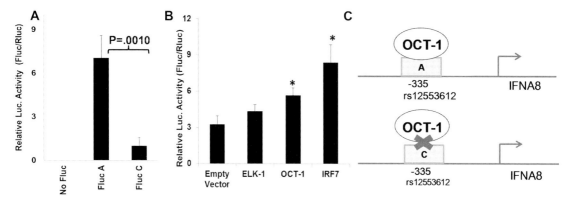

Figure 2. Interferon (IFN)-A8 promoter activity with the A-genotype at –335 is superior to that with the C-genotype. (A) THP-1 cells (1×10^5) were cotransfected with 0.02 µg of pGL4 vector encoding *Renilla luciferase (Rluc)* as internal control and 0.18 µg of pGL4 vector encoding Firefly luciferase downstream of *IFNA8* promoter with A- or C-genotype *(A-Fluc and C-Fluc)*. Twenty-four hours after the cotransfection, luc activity was measured from triplicate cell-lysates, and relative luciferase was calculated (Fluc/Rluc). (B) THP-1 cells were transfected with the A-genotype Fluc-reporter plasmid and the internal control Rluc plasmid, as well as an expression plasmid encoding ELK-1, OCT-1, or IRF-7 as a positive control. Relative luciferase was calculated as Fluc/Rluc. Results are from one of two experiments with similar results. *The values were statistically different ($P < 0.05$) from the control samples with the empty vector by unpaired two-tailed Student's *t*-test. Error bars indicate standard deviation among triplicate sample. OCT-1 transfection did not enhance the activity of the C-genotype Fluc-reporter (shown in the full paper). (C) Schematic demonstration of the OCT-1 binding ability to the *IFNA8* promoter region containing the rs12553612 SNP. Reproduced, with permission, from Ref. 38.

cell line, which demonstrated superior promoter activity of the A-allele compared with the C-allele (Fig. 2A).[38] We then used electrophoretic mobility shift assays to demonstrate that the A-genotype specifically binds to more nuclear proteins than the C-genotype, including the transcription factor Oct-1.[38] When we cotransfected plasmids encoding Oct-1 and the reporter constructs, we observed that Oct-1 enhanced the promoter activity with the A- but not the C-allele (Fig. 2B; shown only for the A-allele).[38] Taken together, our data demonstrate that the A-allele in the rs12553612 SNP, which is associated with better patient survival, allows for *IFNA8* transcription via Oct-1 binding, absent in patients with the C-allele (Fig. 2C),[38] and suggests a molecular mechanism for IFNA8-mediated immunesurveillance of glioma progression.

COX-2 blockade suppresses gliomagenesis: inhibition of immature myeloid cells

Epidemiological findings led to the discovery of key mechanisms and insights contributing to the development of therapeutic and prophylactic strategies. Specifically, based on epidemiological observations[28,29] that chronic use of NSAIDs is associated with reduced risk of glioma,[17,28,29] we translated these findings back to a novel *de novo* glioma model[37] and found that cyclooxygenase (COX)-2 inhibition enhances antiglioma immunosurveillance by reducing glioma-associated myeloid cells.[39] COX-2 and its product prostaglandin E $(PGE)_2$ are known to promote tumor growth and immune escape of tumors through a variety of mechanisms, including the differentiation of Gr-1^+ $CD11b^+$ immunosuppressive IMCs from bone marrow stem cells.[40] Furthermore, PGE_2 produced by the tumor induces arginase 1 and cationic amino acid transporter (CAT)-2B in IMCs, both of which deplete arginine from the tumor microenvironment and impair T cell function.[41,42] Data from the *de novo* glioma model demonstrate that treatment with the COX-2 inhibitors acetylsalicylic acid (ASA) or celecoxib inhibited systemic PGE_2 production and delayed glioma development.[39] ASA treatment also reduced monocyte chemoattracting protein-1, also known as CCL2 (C-C motif ligand 2), in the glioma as well as the number of IMCs in both bone marrow and the glioma. Both ASA-treated and $Cox2^{-/-}$ mice demonstrated a reduction in IMCs and their CCL2-mediated accumulation in the glioma. Conversely, $Cox2^{-/-}$ mice and ASA-treated wild-type mice displayed enhanced expression of CXCL10 (C-X-C motif chemokine 10) and tumor infiltration of cytotoxic T lymphocytes (CTLs).[39]

Although these findings suggest that COX-2 inhibition may be applied to the prevention of gliomas, the use of COX-2 inhibitors, such as celecoxib, to prevent glioma may not be justifiable in the general population due to the increased risk of cardiovascular sequelae[43] and gastrointestinal hemorrhage.[44] However, their use may be justified in populations with a high risk for the development of malignant glioma, such as in patients with LGGs, given their extremely high risk for progression to HGGs. Indeed, the use of celecoxib has been approved by the U.S. Food and Drug Adminstration (FDA) for the prevention of colon cancer in patients with familial adenomatous polyposis. In HGG patients, the use of COX-2 inhibitors has been investigated in combination with retinoids,[45] chemotherapy,[46] and irinotecan[47] regimens that were well tolerated. Although these studies show only modest therapeutic activity in HGG patients, their results provide a basis on which to evaluate the use of COX-2 inhibitors in patients with LGGs, especially in combination with active immunotherapy approaches, such as vaccines, as discussed in more detail in the following section.

Perspective

We next aim to identify new genetic risk and prognostic factors that are supported by an in-depth understanding of their biological mechanisms gained through bench and clinical studies conducted in parallel. Such discoveries could lead to the development and rapid translation of more proactive and personalized treatments (e.g., prophylactic vaccines and/or use of NSAIDs in high-risk populations and/or patients). Further, this work could advance understanding of the immune response characteristics of specific patient groups (e.g., patients with the AC-genotype in the SNP rs12553612 may have suboptimal IFN-α responses), thus allowing selection of more appropriate treatment options for each patient.

Although we still know very little about glioma risk factors, as discussed earlier, we have identified patients with WHO grade II LGGs as a population with a premalignant condition at extremely high risk ($>50\%$) for recurrence as HGGs,[11,12,48,49] and in whom we can test novel preventive therapeutics. Immunotherapeutic modalities, such as vaccines, may offer safe and effective treatment options for these patients due to the slower growth rate

of LGGs (in contrast to HGGs), which should allow sufficient time for multiple immunizations, and hence high levels of antiglioma immunity. Because patients with LGGs are likely not to be as immunocompromised as patients with HGGs, they may exhibit greater immunological response to and benefit from the vaccines. Further, the generally mild toxicity of vaccines may help maintain a higher quality of life than is experienced with current cancer therapy. Indeed, based on encouraging data from a phase I vaccine trial targeting multiple glioma-associated antigen (GAA) epitopes in patients with recurrent HGGs,[50] we have initiated a pilot study of subcutaneous vaccinations with synthetic peptides for GAA epitopes emulsified in Montanide-ISA-51 every 3 weeks for eight courses as well as intramuscular administration of polyICLC[51,52] in human leukocyte antigen (HLA)-A2$^+$ patients with LGGs. Primary endpoints are safety and CD8$^+$ T cell responses against vaccine-targeted GAAs, assessed by enzyme-linked immuno-SPOT (ELISPOT) assays. Treatment response is evaluated clinically and by magnetic resonance imaging (MRI). GAAs for these peptides are IL-13Rα2,[53,54] EphA2,[55] Wilms' tumor gene product 1 (*WT1*),[56,57] and Survivin.[58,59] As these GAAs are expressed in both LGGs and HGGs,[55,57,58,60–63] the regimen used in our pilot study may offer both immunotherapeutic and immunoprophylactic potential to reduce the risk of tumor recurrence. Therapeutically, this approach could suppress the expansion of indolently growing neoplastic LGG cells. Prophylactically, it could prevent the growth of glioma cells that undergo anaplastic transformation. A pan-HLA-DR tetanus toxoid peptide (TetA830) was included to enhance the general helper CD4$^+$ T cell response. To date, 23 patients have been enrolled, and no dose-limiting toxicity has been encountered, except for one case with grade 3 fever (unpublished data). The preliminary results demonstrate that the regimen in these patients is well tolerated and induces a robust type-1 anti-GAA T cell response.

As the time course for LGG patients to recur with HGGs is highly variable and can exceed 10 years, typical funding mechanisms do not support the conclusive evaluation of the efficacy of preventing an LGG to HGG transition. However, due to the challenge of evaluating clinical responses in LGG patients, biomarkers of LGGs are actively being sought.

For example, mutations in *isocitrate dehydrogenases 1* and *2* (*IDH1* and *IDH2*) have been shown to be present in most LGGs,[64] and are associated with the accumulation of 2-hydroxyglutarate (2HG) in the tumor, which can be assessed quantitatively by magnetic resonance spectroscopy,[65] and may thus prove to be a valuable diagnostic and prognostic biomarker in the near future. We will actively incorporate newly available biomarkers that can accurately predict disease progression or recurrence in our future studies. Furthermore, the ultimate success of our vaccine approach will benefit from the blockade of immunosuppressing mechanisms, such as those mediated by IMCs and MDSCs. It will be intriguing to continue to evaluate whether modulation of myeloid cells by clinically available agents, such as celecoxib, will potentiate the effects of glioma vaccines, thereby inhibiting the progression of LGG to HGG.

The studies discussed previously provide unique and privileged opportunities for cooperative synergy and the real-time exchange of data from epidemiologic studies to animal and human studies. In particular, our collective research, conducted in parallel and collaboratively, has identified a critical role for inflammation mediators, such as myeloid cells, in glioma development. These data[30,38,39] demonstrate how epidemiology studies can be driven by preclinical data in highly clinically relevant mouse models (biology-driven epidemiology), and how molecular biology can validate epidemiological findings and delineate the underlying novel mechanisms that could inform the development of therapeutic and/or preventive strategies (epidemiology-driven biology).

Acknowledgments

This work was supported by grants from the National Institutes of Health (K07CA131505, R01CA119215, R01CA070917, R01NS055140, P01NS40923, P01CA132714, and U24AI082673) and the Musella Foundation for Brain Tumor Research and Information. The authors thank Michelle L. Kienholz for her critical review of the manuscript.

Conflicts of interest

Hideho Okada is an inventor of the HLA-A2-binding CTL epitope peptide derived from IL-13Rα2, which has been exclusively licensed to Stemline Therapeutics, Inc. (U.S. Application Serial # 11/231,618), and also serves on the Advisory Board of Stemline Therapeutics, Inc. Hideho Okada has completed all COI management plans according to University of Pittsburgh COI policies. Data related to the use of this invention were not evaluated or interpreted by Hideho Okada alone, but by the entire research team collaboratively.

References

1. CBTRUS. 2012. Statistical report: primary brain and central nervous system tumors diagnosed in the United States in 2004–2008, Central Brain Tumor Registry of the United States.
2. Karim, A.B., B. Maat, R. Hatlevoll, *et al.* 1996. A randomized trial on dose-response in radiation therapy of low-grade cerebral glioma: European Organization for Research and Treatment of Cancer (EORTC) study 22844. *Int. J. Radiat. Oncol. Biol. Phys.* **36:** 549–556.
3. van den Bent, M.J., D. Afra, W.O. De, *et al.* 2005. Long-term efficacy of early versus delayed radiotherapy for low-grade astrocytoma and oligodendroglioma in adults: the EORTC 22845 randomised trial. *Lancet* **366:** 985–990.
4. Karim, A.B., D. Afra, P. Cornu, *et al.* 2002. Randomized trial on the efficacy of radiotherapy for cerebral low-grade glioma in the adult: European Organization for Research and Treatment of Cancer Study 22845 with the Medical Research Council study BRO4: an interim analysis. *Int. J. Radiat. Oncol. Biol. Phys.* **52:** 316–324.
5. Shaw, E., R. Arusell, B. Scheithauer, *et al.* 2002. Prospective randomized trial of low- versus high-dose radiation therapy in adults with supratentorial low-grade glioma: initial report of a North Central Cancer Treatment Group/Radiation Therapy Oncology Group/Eastern Cooperative Oncology Group study. *J. Clin. Oncol.* **20:** 2267–2276.
6. Shaw, E.G., B. Berkey, S.W. Coons, *et al.* 2006. Radiation Therapy Oncology Group Protocol 9802: radiation therapy alone versus RT + PCV chemotherapy in adult low-grade glioma. *Neuro Oncol.* **8:** 489.
7. Shaw, E.G., B. Berkey, S.W. Coons, *et al.* 2006. Update of an RTOG prospective study of observation in completely resected adult low-grade glioma. *Neuro Oncol.* **8:** 452.
8. Papagikos, M.A., E.G. Shaw, & V.W. Stieber. 2005. Lessons learned from randomised clinical trials in adult low-grade glioma. *Lancet Oncol.* **6:** 240–244.
9. Pignatti, F., B.M. van den, D. Curran, *et al.* 2002. Prognostic factors for survival in adult patients with cerebral low-grade glioma. *J. Clin. Oncol.* **20:** 2076–2084.
10. Shaw, E.G., B. Berkey, S.W. Coons, *et al.* 2008. Recurrence following neurosurgeon-determined gross total resection of adult supratentorial low-grade glioma: results of a prospective clinical trial. *J. Neurosurg.* **109:** 835–841.
11. Brown, P.D., E.G. Shaw, L.L. Gunderson, *et al.* 2006. *Low-Grade Gliomas, Clinical Radiation Oncology.* 493–514. Philadelphia, PA: Churchill-Livingstone.
12. Sanai, N., S. Chang & M.S. Berger. 2011. Low-grade gliomas in adults. *J. Neurosurg.* **115:** 948–965.

13. Fisher, J.L., J.A. Schwartzbaum, M. Wrensch, *et al.* 2007. Epidemiology of brain tumors. *Neurol. Clin.* **25**: 867–890.

14. Schwartzbaum, J.A., K. Huang, S. Lawler, *et al.* 2010. Allergy and inflammatory transcriptome is predominantly negatively correlated with CD133 expression in glioblastoma. *Neuro Oncol.* **12**: 320–327.

15. Schwartzbaum, J.A., A. Ahlbom, S. Lonn, *et al.* 2007. An international case-control study of interleukin-4Ralpha, interleukin-13, and cyclooxygenase-2 polymorphisms and glioblastoma risk. *Cancer Epidemiol. Biomarkers Prev.* **16**: 2448–2454.

16. Schwartzbaum, J., A. Ahlbom, B. Malmer, *et al.* 2005. Polymorphisms associated with asthma are inversely related to glioblastoma multiforme. *Cancer Res.* **65**: 6459–6465.

17. Sivak-Sears, N.R., J.A. Schwartzbaum, R. Miike, *et al.* 2004. Case-control study of use of nonsteroidal antiinflammatory drugs and glioblastoma multiforme. *Am. J. Epidemiol.* **159**: 1131–1139.

18. McCarthy, B.J., K.M. Rankin, K. Aldape, *et al.* 2011. Risk factors for oligodendroglial tumors: a pooled international study. *Neuro Oncol.* **13**: 242–250.

19. Schoemaker, M.J., A.J. Swerdlow, S.J. Hepworth, *et al.* 2006. History of allergies and risk of glioma in adults. *Int. J. Cancer* **119**: 2165–2172.

20. Brenner, A.V., M.A. Butler, S.S. Wang, *et al.* 2007. Single-nucleotide polymorphisms in selected cytokine genes and risk of adult glioma. *Carcinogenesis* **28**: 2543–2547.

21. Brenner, A.V., M.S. Linet, H.A. Fine, *et al.* 2002. History of allergies and autoimmune diseases and risk of brain tumors in adults. *Int. J. Cancer* **99**: 252–259.

22. Linos, E., T. Raine, A. Alonso, *et al.* 2007. Atopy and risk of brain tumors: a meta-analysis. *J. Natl. Cancer Instit.* **99**: 1544–1550.

23. Wiemels, J.L., J.K. Wiencke, K.T. Kelsey, *et al.* 2007. Allergy-related polymorphisms influence glioma status and serum IgE levels. *Cancer Epidemiol. Biomarkers Prev.* **16**: 1229–1235.

24. Wiemels, J.L., J.K. Wiencke, J.D. Sison, *et al.* 2002. History of allergies among adults with glioma and controls. *Int. J. Cancer* **98**: 609–615.

25. Wrensch, M., J.K. Wiencke, J. Wiemels, *et al.* 2006. Serum IgE, tumor epidermal growth factor receptor expression, and inherited polymorphisms associated with glioma survival. *Cancer Res.* **66**: 4531–4541.

26. Schwartzbaum, J.A., J.L. Fisher, K.D. Aldape, *et al.* 2006. Epidemiology and molecular pathology of glioma. *Nat. Clin. Pract. Neurol.* **2**: 494–503.

27. Scheurer, M.E., E. Amirian, Y. Cao, *et al.* 2008. Polymorphisms in the interleukin-4 receptor gene are associated with better survival in patients with glioblastoma. *Clin. Cancer Res.* **14**: 6640–6646.

28. Scheurer, M.E., E.S. Amirian, S.L. Davlin, *et al.* 2011. Effects of antihistamine and anti-inflammatory medication use on risk of specific glioma histologies. *Int. J. Cancer* **129**: 2290–2296.

29. Scheurer, M.E., R. El-Zein, P.A. Thompson, *et al.* 2008. Long-term anti-inflammatory and antihistamine medication use and adult glioma risk. *Cancer Epidemiol. Biomarkers Prev.* **17**: 1277–1281.

30. Fujita, M., M.E. Scheurer, S.A. Decker, *et al.* 2010. Role of type 1 IFNs in antiglioma immunosurveillance—using mouse studies to guide examination of novel prognostic markers in humans. *Clin. Cancer Res.* **16**: 3409–3419.

31. Schwartzbaum, J.A., Y. Xiao, Y. Liu, *et al.* 2010. Inherited variation in immune genes and pathways and glioblastoma risk. *Carcinogenesis* **31**: 1770–1777.

32. Amirian, E., Y. Liu, M.E. Scheurer, *et al.* 2010. Genetic variants in inflammation pathway genes and asthma in glioma susceptibility. *Neuro Oncol.* **12**: 444–452.

33. Nakahara, N., I.F. Pollack, W.J. Storkus, *et al.* 2003. Effective induction of antiglioma cytotoxic T cells by coadministration of interferon-beta gene vector and dendritic cells. *Cancer Gene Ther.* **10**: 549–558.

34. Tsugawa, T., N. Kuwashima, H. Sato, *et al.* 2004. Sequential delivery of interferon-gene and DCs to intracranial gliomas promotes an effective anti-tumor response. *Gene Ther.* **11**: 1551–1558.

35. Kuwashima, N., F. Nishimura, J. Eguchi, *et al.* 2005. Delivery of dendritic cells engineered to secrete IFN-alpha into central nervous system tumors enhances the efficacy of peripheral tumor cell vaccines: dependence on apoptotic pathways. *J. Immunol.* **175**: 2730–2740.

36. Nishimura, F., J.E. Dusak, J. Eguchi, *et al.* 2006. Adoptive transfer of Type 1 CTL mediates effective anti-central nervous system tumor response: critical roles of IFN-inducible protein-10. *Cancer Res.* **66**: 4478–4487.

37. Wiesner, S.M., S.A. Decker, J.D. Larson, *et al.* 2009. De novo induction of genetically engineered brain tumors in mice using plasmid DNA. *Cancer Res.* **69**: 431–439.

38. Kohanbash, G., E. Ishikawa, M. Fujita, *et al.* 2012. Differential activity of interferon-α8 promoter is regulated by Oct-1 and a SNP that dictates prognosis of glioma. *OncoImmunology* **1**: 487–492.

39. Fujita, M., G. Kohanbash, W. Fellows-Mayle, *et al.* 2011. COX-2 blockade suppresses gliomagenesis by inhibiting myeloid-derived suppressor cells. *Cancer Res.* **71**: 2664–2674.

40. Sinha, P., V.K. Clements, A.M. Fulton, *et al.* 2007. Prostaglandin E2 promotes tumor progression by inducing myeloid-derived suppressor cells. *Cancer Res.* **67**: 4507–4513.

41. Ochoa, A.C., A.H. Zea, C. Hernandez, *et al.* 2007. Arginase, prostaglandins, and myeloid-derived suppressor cells in renal cell carcinoma. *Clin. Cancer Res.* **13**: 721s–726s.

42. Rodriguez, P.C. & A.C. Ochoa. 2008. Arginine regulation by myeloid derived suppressor cells and tolerance in cancer: mechanisms and therapeutic perspectives. *Immunol. Rev.* **222**: 180–191.

43. Solomon, S.D., J. Wittes, P.V. Finn, *et al.* 2008. Cardiovascular risk of celecoxib in 6 randomized placebo-controlled trials: the cross trial safety analysis. *Circulation* **117**: 2104–2113.

44. Fidler, M.J., A. Argiris, J.D. Patel, *et al.* 2008. The potential predictive value of cyclooxygenase-2 expression and increased risk of gastrointestinal hemorrhage in advanced non-small cell lung cancer patients treated with erlotinib and celecoxib. *Clin. Cancer Res.* **14**: 2088–2094.

45. Giglio, P. & V. Levin. 2004. Cyclooxygenase-2 inhibitors in glioma therapy. *Am. J. Ther.* **11**: 141–143.

46. Hau, P., L. Kunz-Schughart, U. Bogdahn, *et al.* 2007. Low-dose chemotherapy in combination with COX-2 inhibitors and PPAR-gamma agonists in recurrent high-grade gliomas—a phase II study. *Oncology* **73:** 21–25.

47. Reardon, D.A., J.A. Quinn, J. Vredenburgh, *et al.* 2005. Phase II trial of irinotecan plus celecoxib in adults with recurrent malignant glioma. *Cancer* **103:** 329–338.

48. Baumert, B.G. & R. Stupp. 2008. Low-grade glioma: a challenge in therapeutic options: the role of radiotherapy. *Ann. Oncol.* **19:** vii217–vii222.

49. Ashby, L.S. & W.R. Shapiro. 2004. Low-grade glioma: supratentorial astrocytoma, oligodendroglioma, and oligoastrocytoma in adults. *Curr. Neurol. Neurosci. Rep.* **4:** 211–217.

50. Okada, H., P. Kalinski, R. Ueda, *et al.* 2011. Induction of CD8[+] T-cell responses against novel glioma-associated antigen peptides and clinical activity by vaccinations with {alpha}-type 1 polarized dendritic cells and polyinosinic-polycytidylic acid stabilized by lysine and carboxymethylcellulose in patients with recurrent malignant glioma. *J. Clin. Oncol.* **29:** 330–336.

51. Zhu, X., B. Fallert-Junecko, M. Fujita, *et al.* 2010. Poly-ICLC promotes the infiltration of effector T cells into intracranial gliomas via induction of CXCL10 in IFN-α and IFN-γ dependent manners. *Cancer Immunol. Immunother.* **59:** 1401–1409.

52. Zhu, X., F. Nishimura, K. Sasaki, *et al.* 2007. Toll-like receptor-3 ligand poly-ICLC promotes the efficacy of peripheral vaccinations with tumor antigen-derived peptide epitopes in murine CNS tumor models. *J. Transl. Med.* **5:** 10.

53. Eguchi, J., M. Hatano, F. Nishimura, *et al.* 2006. Identification of interleukin-13 receptor alpha2 peptide analogues capable of inducing improved antiglioma CTL responses. *Cancer Res.* **66:** 5883–5891.

54. Okano, F., W.J. Storkus, W.H. Chambers, *et al.* 2002. Identification of a novel HLA-A*0201 restricted cytotoxic T lymphocyte epitope in a human glioma associated antigen, interleukin-13 receptor 2 chain. *Clin. Cancer Res.* **8:** 2851–2855.

55. Hatano, M., J. Eguchi, T. Tatsumi, *et al.* 2005. EphA2 as a glioma-associated antigen: a novel target for glioma vaccines. *Neoplasia* **7:** 717–722.

56. Al Qudaihi, G., C. Lehe, M. Negash, *et al.* 2009. Enhancement of lytic activity of leukemic cells by CD8[+] cytotoxic T lymphocytes generated against a WT1 peptide analogue. *Leukemia Lymphoma* **50:** 260–269.

57. Nakahara, Y., H. Okamoto, T. Mineta, *et al.* 2004. Expression of the Wilms' tumor gene product WT1 in glioblastomas and medulloblastomas. *Brain Tumor Pathol.* **21:** 113–116.

58. Uematsu, M., I. Ohsawa, T. Aokage, *et al.* 2005. Prognostic significance of the immunohistochemical index of survivin in glioma: a comparative study with the MIB-1 index. *J. Neurooncol.* **72:** 231–238.

59. Andersen, M.H., L.O. Pedersen, J.C. Becker, *et al.* 2001. Identification of a cytotoxic T lymphocyte response to the apoptosis inhibitor protein survivin in cancer patients. *Cancer Res.* **61:** 869–872.

60. Ciesielski, M., D. Kozbor, C. Castanaro, *et al.* 2008. Therapeutic effect of a T helper cell supported CTL response induced by a survivin peptide vaccine against murine cerebral glioma. *Cancer Immunol. Immunother.* **57:** 1827–1835.

61. Debinski, W. & D.M. Gibo. 2000. Molecular expression analysis of restrictive receptor for interleukin 13, a brain tumor-associated cancer/testis antigen. *Mol. Med.* **6:** 440–449.

62. Debinski, W., D.M. Gibo, S.W. Hulet, *et al.* 1999. Receptor for interleukin 13 is a marker and therapeutic target for human high-grade gliomas. *Clin. Cancer Res.* **5:** 985–990.

63. Wykosky, J., D.M. Gibo, C. Stanton, *et al.* 2005. EphA2 as a novel molecular marker and target in glioblastoma multiforme. *Mol. Cancer Res.* **3:** 541–551.

64. Yan, H., D.W. Parsons, G. Jin, *et al.* 2009. IDH1 and IDH2 mutations in gliomas. *N. Engl. J. Med.* **360:** 765–773.

65. Choi, C., S.K. Ganji, R.J. DeBerardinis, *et al.* 2012. 2-hydroxyglutarate detection by magnetic resonance spectroscopy in IDH-mutated patients with gliomas. *Nat. Med.* **18:** 624–629.

Ann. N.Y. Acad. Sci. ISSN 0077-8923

Human dendritic cells subsets as targets and vectors for therapy

Eynav Klechevsky[1] and Jacques Banchereau[2]

[1]Department of Pathology and Immunology, Washington University School of Medicine, St. Louis, Missouri.
[2]jacques. banchereau@gmail.com

Address for correspondence: Eynav Klechevsky, Department of Pathology and Immunology, Washington University School of Medicine, St. Louis, MO 63110. eklechevsky@path.wustl.edu

The skin immune system includes a complex network of dendritic cells (DCs). In addition to generating cellular and humoral immunity against pathogens, skin DCs are involved in tolerogenic mechanisms that maintain immune homeostasis and in pathogenic chronic inflammation in which immune responses are unrestrained. Harnessing DC function by directly targeting DC-derived molecules or by selectively modulating DC subsets is a novel strategy for ameliorating inflammatory diseases. In this short review, we discuss recent advances in understanding the functional specialization of skin DCs and the potential implication for future DC-based therapeutic strategies.

Keywords: dendritic cells; human DCs; skin; inflammation; therapy

Introduction

Ralph Steinman identified dendritic cells (DCs) in 1973 as an accessory cell type of the mouse spleen. Studies of the past two decades have established that, both in mice and humans, DCs comprise subsets that differ in localization, phenotype, and some functions, while also having common properties. Human skin contains several distinct DC subsets.

During the past 20 years, we have focused on DC subsets, including early studies on DCs generated *in vitro*[1,2] that revealed similarities and differences among the various DC types. Human DCs generated by culturing CD34[+] hematopoietic progenitor cells with a combination of granulocyte-macrophage colony-stimulating factor (GM-CSF), TNF-α, and FLT-3 ligand, for example, include CD1a- and CD14-expressing subsets that have unique phenotypes, cytokine secretion potential, and function. As CD14[+], but not CD1a[+], DCs can directly prime activated naive B cells in IgM-secreting plasma cells. More recently, our focus has been on human skin DC subsets. The epidermis contains Langerhans cells (LCs) and the dermis has at least three subsets, CD1a[+], CD14[+], and CD141[+] DCs, in addition to skin-resident macrophages.[3]

Here, we summarize what we have learned and reported in several papers,[4–7] particularly as it relates to the control of CD8[+] T cell (CTL) responses. We also integrate our data within the context of studies performed by other groups in the field.

DC subsets in human skin

Epidermal LCs and dermal CD14[+] DCs have phenotypic and functional differences. Dermal CD14[+] DCs express a large number of C-type lectins, including DC-SIGN (dendritic cell-specific intercellular adhesion molecule-3-grabbing nonintegrin), LOX-1 (lectin-like oxidized LDL receptor-1), CLEC-6 (C-type lectin domain family 1 member-6), dectin-1, and DCIR (dendritic cell immunoreceptor)/CLEC4A, while LCs express langerin/CD207, DEC205/CD205, and DCIR/CLEC4A. Dermal CD14[+] DCs also express Toll-like receptors (TLRs), such as TLR2, 4, 5, 6, 8, and 10, that are specific for bacterial pathogen-associated molecular patterns (PAMPs);[6,8] LCs express fewer TLRs, including TLR1, 2, 3, 6, and 10.[8,9]

LCs and CD14[+] DCs produce different cytokines upon stimulation via CD40. CD14[+] DCs produce IL-1α, IL-6, IL-8, IL-10, IL-12, GM-CSF, MCP-1/CCL2, and TGF-β, while LCs produce only a few cytokines, including IL-15.[4] Such cytokine production differences appear to explain, at least in part, why the two subsets induce adaptive immune

doi: 10.1111/nyas.12113

responses with different qualities, as will be discussed below.

In addition, human skin contains a population of CD141-expressing cells, which also express cell surface markers that are expressed by the mouse CD8α^+ DCs and have the capacity to cross-present antigens to CD8$^+$ T cells (see Ref. 10 and unpublished data from Klechevsky's laboratory). Thus, human skin harbors an array of DC subsets with shared, as well as unique, characteristics.

Langerhans cells efficiently induce CD8$^+$ T cell responses through IL-15

We found that epidermal CD1a$^+$ langerin$^+$ LCs and dermal CD14$^+$ DCs have the potential to stimulate different types of adaptive immunity. While LCs are efficient at inducing CTL responses, CD14$^+$ dermal DCs display the unique property of promoting the development of antibody responses, either by directly acting on activated B cells or by priming T follicular helper (T$_{FH}$)-like CD4$^+$ T cells. The dermis contains a DC population that expresses CD1a but not langerin and displays functions of both LCs and CD14$^+$ DCs, although to a lesser extent. Considering that the two DC subsets—LCs and CD14$^+$ DCs—produce distinct cytokines, we examined the role of the subset-specific cytokines IL-15 and IL-10, respectively, in inducing CD8$^+$ T cell responses.

Results from four complementary experimental approaches enabled us to conclude that the production of IL-15 by LCs is critical for promoting differentiation of naive CD8$^+$ T cells into granzyme B$^+$ perforin$^+$ CTLs.

First, LCs, but not CD14$^+$ DCs, transcribe and secrete IL-15, which binds to its receptor at the interface between LCs and CD8$^+$ T cells. CD1a$^+$ dermal DCs, which are intermediate activators of CD8$^+$ naive T cells,[6] also transcribe IL-15.

Second, addition of neutralizing antibodies to IL-15 (and its receptor) partially inhibits LC-mediated differentiation of naive CD8$^+$ T cells to effector CTLs.

Third, addition of IL-15 to cocultures of naive CD8$^+$ T cells and dermal CD14$^+$ DCs enhanced, in a dose-dependent manner, their ability to prime effector CD8$^+$ T cells. The CD8$^+$ T cells primed by dermal CD14$^+$ DCs and IL-15 showed an increased effector phenotype, as measured by the level of granzymes, CD25, CCR7, and CD28, which are comparable to the levels observed by LC-primed CD8$^+$ T cells. Expression of the anti-apoptotic molecule Bcl-2 was also elevated in CD8$^+$ T cells upon priming with dermal CD14$^+$ DCs and IL-15; this finding is consistent with observations in the mouse that IL-15 increases Bcl-2 expression in antigen-induced CD8$^+$ T cells.[11]

Fourth, immunofluorescence studies using confocal microscopy indicated that IL-15 is being secreted directly into the immunological synapses between naive CD8$^+$ T cells and LCs and dermal CD1a$^+$ DCs.

Studies from other groups are consistent with our findings on the role of DC-derived IL-15 in the induction of potent CTL responses *in vitro* and *in vivo*, in both mouse and human.[12–14] Thus, the capacity of LCs to initiate CD8$^+$ T cell immunity highlights the important role of IL-15 produced by LCs; in contrast, as will be discussed below, a regulatory role has been shown for IL-10 produced by dermal CD14$^+$ DCs.

Dermal CD14$^+$ DC–derived IL-10 limits CTL priming and induces T$_{reg}$ cells

The CTL responses induced by CD14$^+$ dermal DCs are less potent than those induced by LCs. In addition, CD4$^+$ T cells primed by CD14$^+$ DCs are unique in their ability to promote the development of antibody responses, either directly or by priming T$_{FH}$-like CD4$^+$ T cells. IL-12 produced by dermal CD14$^+$ DCs, but not LCs, is a key cytokine in priming this response.[15–17] CD14$^+$ dermal DCs also secrete large amounts of IL-10.[4] IL-10 has broad anti-inflammatory properties, acting on both T cells[18] and antigen-presenting cells.[20] In particular, IL-10 prevents CD8$^+$ T cells from upregulating the effector molecules granzyme and perforin. TGF-β1 also contributes to the specific effects of CD14$^+$ DCs on CD8$^+$ T-cell differentiation;[21] for example, TGF-β1 delivers an extrinsic signal in opposition to IL-15 to control the number of short-lived effector cells during clonal expansion and contraction during viral infection.[11,22] TGF-β1 functions in synergy with IL-10 to inhibit both proliferation and effector molecule production by CD8$^+$ T cells primed by LCs. CD14$^+$ DCs, but not LCs, transcribe TGF-β1,[4] although TGF-β1 protein is not measurable in DC supernatants ELISA assay. It might be secreted by the dermal CD14$^+$ DCs at very low (undetectable by ELISA) levels[4] that are nevertheless sufficient to enhance the regulatory effects of IL-10.

In sum, LCs and dermal CD1a[+] DCs present IL-15 to naive CD8[+] T cells at the immunological synapse, resulting in potent CTL priming. In opposition to this activity, dermal CD14[+] DCs express IL-10 and TGF-β1, but not IL-15, which prevents the generation of effector CD8[+] T cells. These findings have several clinical implications, including that inhibition of IL-10 and TGF-β1 signaling may help to overcome tumor resistance and improve the potency of tumor immunotherapy.[17,23–25]

Our findings with human cells support these studies, and further provide a cellular mechanism by which blocking IL-10 and TGF-β signaling results in enhanced effector responses. In addition, the efficacy of IL-15 in eradicating tumors through enhanced induction of functional CD8[+] cytotoxic T cells has been well documented in mouse tumor models.[26,27] The delivery of antigen to IL-15–producing LCs for induction of therapeutic antigen-specific CTL responses, as well as generating DC vaccines using IL-15 as an adjuvant, are also supported.

Related to this, it will be interesting to determine the extent to which DCs that infiltrate various tumors possess properties of immune-suppressing dermal CD14[+] DCs. We and others have shown that infiltration of certain tumors with DCs induces T cell differentiation along the Th2 pathway.[28,29] However, tumors may also be infiltrated by DCs with the properties of dermal CD14[+] DCs, which would skew differentiation of CD8[+] T cells into noncytolytic T cells (and hence unable to kill tumor cells).[30]

Dermal CD14[+] DC ILT receptors prevent efficient CTL priming

Our detailed phenotypic analysis has shown that naive CD8[+] T cells primed with LCs generate CD8[hi], poly-functional T cells, while those primed with dermal CD14[+] DCs display lower levels of surface CD8 and have less killing activity. Naive CD8[+] T cells primed with CD14[+] DCs produce type 2–associated cytokines (IL-4, IL-5, and IL-13) and are associated with a lower frequency of granzyme- and perforin-expressing cells, lower expression of surface CD8 and CD25, and higher expression of CD30 and CD40L.[31–33]

We have found that stimulation of naive CD8[+] T cells with TGF-β and IL-10 alone only partially reproduces these phenotypes, which suggests that der-

mal CD14[+] DCs might also express a cell-intrinsic factor that blocks CD8 function. In addition, in separate studies, allogeneic response studies with LCs using an anti-CD8 mAb that limits CD8 density on naive T cells resulted in diminished T cell proliferation and quality; in particular, the CD8[+] T cells displayed a TC2 phenotype associated with a lower frequency of granzyme- and perforin-expressing cells, and lower expression of surface CD8 and CD25, but higher levels of CD30 and CD40L.[31–33]

On the basis of that work, we performed transcriptomic analysis and found that dermal CD14[+] DCs express Ig-like transcript 4 (ILT4) and ILT2, known inhibitors of CD8 binding to major histocompatibility complex (MHC) class I;[34–36] structural modeling demonstrated that ILT2 and ILT4 sterically interfere with CD8 binding to MHC class I. ILT receptors impair NK cell function and promote the generation of regulatory CD8[+] and CD4[+] T cells.[37] The mouse homolog PIR-B also regulates the suppressive function of myeloid-derived suppressor cells.[38] Introducing soluble ILT fusion proteins to cocultures of LCs and naive CD8[+] T cells, and blocking ILT receptors on dermal CD14[+] DCs using anti-ILT antibodies, allowed us to demonstrate that ILT4 and, to a lesser extent, ILT2 regulate the generation of effector CD8[+] T cells by dermal CD14[+] DCs.

The biological role of type 2–polarized CD8[+] T cells (TC2 cells) remains poorly understood. An early study showed that IL-4 produced by CD8[+] T suppressor clones from immunologically unresponsive individuals with leprosy was necessary for suppression observed in vitro.[39] Patient studies have shown expansion of TC2 populations in various disease conditions, including cancer[40–42] and chronic viral infections;[32,43] in these cases, TC2 accumulation appeared to be associated with disease pathogenesis. In addition, CD40L- and IL-4–producing CD8[+] T (TC2) cells have B cell helper functions[32,44,45] (which is consistent with our proposed role of CD14[+] DCs in the control of humoral responses).[2,4] Given the above, blocking CD8 may have potential clinical applications, such as controlling the pathogenic effect of allogeneic CD8[+] T cells in allograft rejection; this would still allow for productive, specific recall responses, in contrast with nonspecific immunosuppressive therapies that increase susceptibility to viral infections.

Thus, CD8 modulation during a primary response is a mechanism for regulating the balance between type 1 effector and type 2 suppressive responses. Our data suggest that, by expressing the inhibitory receptors ILT2 and ILT4, dermal CD14[+] DCs block efficient CTL differentiation and instead enhance the generation of TC2 cells. This complements an elegant study from another group demonstrating that the dermal CD14[+] DCs prime T_{reg} cells in a skin-transplanted mouse model.[46]

Looking beyond those results, viruses such as cytomegalovirus (CMV) that express class-I–like proteins[47] might use this mechanism to inhibit induction of viral-specific CD8[+] T cells and to promote TC2 cell responses that have only a limited ability to clear infected or malignant cells. Similarly, tumors might upregulate surface ILT2 or ILT4 to attenuate the production of CTLs. Strategies to block ILT expression on DCs may help augment dendritic cell function and enhance immune responses to chronic viral infections and cancer. Alternatively, mobilizing dermal CD14[+] DCs may be a useful approach to attenuate effector responses in order to combat transplant rejection and chronic inflammatory diseases.

CD141 DCs

While clear characterization of similarities among human and mouse DC subsets was hampered by differences in surface marker expression and by the use of different tissues as a source of DCs, recent broad and unbiased genomic approaches have allowed a better comparison.

Analyses of human blood and mouse spleen DC subsets[48] have shown that human DCs expressing high CD141 (BDCA3) are equivalent in function to mouse CD8α-type DCs.[49–52] Markers conserved across species for these cell types have been identified and include, in particular, the endocytic C-type lectin receptor CLEC9A[53,54] and the chemokine receptor XCR.[50,51] The above analyses predicted that CD11c[hi] CD1a[+] CD141[hi] CLEC9A[+] TLR3[+] DCs would be the professional cross-presenting subtype in humans.[55] Indeed, it was demonstrated that blood CD141[+] DCs are specialized to activate CD8[+] T lymphocytes and to produce IL-12p70 more efficiently than the other DC subsets, similar to mouse CD8α[+] DCs. In addition, cells with similar features can be found in skin dermis, lung, and liver in humans,[10] and might be the equivalent of the der-

mal mouse CD103[+] DCs. However, as all features of the mouse CD103[+] DCs are not conserved in a single human DC subset,[10,46,56] additional studies are required to rigorously establish this point.

Avenues to improve and make new vaccines

Targeting DC subsets in vivo

Specifically targeting DCs represents a vaccine approach to deliver antigens directly to these cells *in vivo*; for example, one approach has used chimeric proteins composed of an anti-DC receptor antibody and an antigen. Pioneering studies by Michel Nussenzweig and Ralph Steinman using antibodies directed to the DC receptor DEC205 demonstrated that targeting antigens to DCs via DEC205 *in vivo* results in a potent induction of antigen-specific CD4[+] and CD8[+] T cells, provided adjuvants are coadministered to activate the targeted DCs.[57,58] The same group also elegantly proved *in vivo* that distinct DC subsets differentially regulate T cell immunity.[59]

Our own studies with human skin DC subsets suggest that LCs are potential targets for inducing potent antigen-specific CTL responses. Indeed, LCs targeted with a fusion protein composed of anti-DCIR antibody conjugated with antigen efficiently cross-present to CD8[+] T cells and thereby induces their proliferation *in vitro*.[60] Similar findings were also obtained when LCs were targeted with anti-Langerin antibody.[60] Furthermore, mouse studies demonstrated that injection of anti-Langerin chimeric proteins induces antigen-specific CD4[+] and CD8[+] T cell responses *in vivo*.[61] These observations provide a rationale for targeting antigens to LCs for CTL responses.

Likewise, CLEC9A might represent an interesting molecule to target blood CD141[+] DCs that are cross-presenters. The means to specifically target skin CD141[hi] DCs, rather than the regulatory dermal CD14[+] DCs that also express CD141, need to be identified. Studies in mice have shown that targeting antigen to CLEC9A[+] cells *in vivo* results in potent cytotoxic T lymphocyte responses, when targeting is combined with anti-CD40 administration,[62] and potent antibody responses, even without coadministration of adjuvants.[53]

Combination therapy

Hopefully, improved vaccines will complement other antitumor approaches, such as checkpoint blockade with anti-CTLA-4 or anti-PD1, which aim to block immune evasion mechanisms such as T_{reg} and myeloid-derived suppressor cell activity in tumors or secretion of suppressive cytokines. Indeed, recent evidence in phase III studies of patients with cancer indicates that vaccination coupled with direct T cell intervention via anti-CTLA-4 blockade has clinical benefit.[63] Tumors might also upregulate surface ILT2 or ILT4 to attenuate the production of CTLs. Strategies to block ILT expression on DCs may thus be useful for augmenting dendritic cell function in order to enhance immune responses to chronic viral infections and cancer.

Concluding remarks and acknowledgments

We dedicate this review to our dear friend and colleague Ralph Steinman, who was awarded the Nobel Prize in 2011 for discovering the dendritic cell and its role in adaptive immunity. Ralph used his own dendritic cells to treat his cancer, which he believed greatly extended his life. He recognized that eliciting T cell immunity in humans is challenging but deserves further exploration. Ralph always urged scientists (young and experienced) with talent for working with DCs and for other areas of immunology to collaborate in order to provide an immune-specific arm to cancer treatment. We are left inspired and highly motivated to continue his legacy.

We thank all of the patients and volunteers who participated in our studies and clinical trials. We also thank former and current members of Baylor Institute for Immunology Research, Washington University School of Medicine, and Barnes Jewish Hospital in St. Louis for their contributions, particularly H. Ueno, J. Fay, A.K. Palucka, G. Zurawski, A. Shaw, M. Colonna, M. Cella, and R. Schreiber.

Conflicts of interest

The authors declare no conflicts of interest.

References

1. Caux, C. et al. 1996. CD34+ hematopoietic progenitors from human cord blood differentiate along two independent dendritic cell pathways in response to GM-CSF+TNF alpha. J. Exp. Med. 184: 695–706.

2. Caux, C. et al. 1997. CD34+ hematopoietic progenitors from human cord blood differentiate along two independent dendritic cell pathways in response to granulocyte-macrophage colony-stimulating factor plus tumor necrosis factor alpha. II: functional analysis. Blood 90: 1458–1470.

3. Valladeau, J. & S. Saeland. 2005. Cutaneous dendritic cells. Semin. Immunol. 17: 273–283.

4. Klechevsky, E. et al. 2008. Functional specializations of human epidermal Langerhans cells and CD14+ dermal dendritic cells. Immunity 29: 497–510.

5. Banchereau, J. et al. 2012. The differential production of cytokines by human Langerhans cells and dermal CD14(+) DCs controls CTL priming. Blood 119: 5742–5749.

6. Klechevsky, E. et al. 2009. Understanding human myeloid dendritic cell subsets for the rational design of novel vaccines. Hum. Immunol. 70: 281–288.

7. Banchereau, J. et al. 2012. Immunoglobulin-like transcript receptors on human dermal CD14+ dendritic cells act as a CD8-antagonist to control cytotoxic T cell priming. Proc. Natl. Acad. Sci. USA 109: 18885–18890.

8. van der Aar, A.M. et al. 2007. Loss of TLR2, TLR4, and TLR5 on Langerhans cells abolishes bacterial recognition. J. Immunol. 178: 1986–1990.

9. Flacher, V. et al. 2006. Human Langerhans cells express a specific TLR profile and differentially respond to viruses and Gram-positive bacteria. J. Immunol. 177: 7959–7967.

10. Haniffa, M. et al. 2012. Human tissues contain CD141hi cross-presenting dendritic cells with functional homology to mouse CD103+ nonlymphoid dendritic cells. Immunity 37: 60–73.

11. Sanjabi, S., M.M. Mosaheb & R.A. Flavell. 2009. Opposing effects of TGF-beta and IL-15 cytokines control the number of short-lived effector CD8+ T cells. Immunity 31: 131–144.

12. Ruckert, R. et al. 2003. Dendritic cell-derived IL-15 controls the induction of CD8 T cell immune responses. Eur. J. Immunol. 33: 3493–3503.

13. Romano, E. et al. 2012. Human Langerhans cells use IL-15Rα/IL-15/pSTAT5-dependent mechanism to break T-cell tolerance against the self-differentiation tumor antigen WT1. Blood 116: 5182–5190.

14. Romano, E. et al. 2011. Peptide-loaded Langerhans cells, despite increased IL15 secretion and T-cell activation in vitro, elicit antitumor T-cell responses comparable to peptide-loaded monocyte-derived dendritic cells in vivo. Clin. Cancer Res. 17: 1984–1997.

15. Dubois, B. et al. 1998. Critical role of IL-12 in dendritic cell-induced differentiation of naive B lymphocytes. J. Immunol. 161: 2223–2231.

16. Schmitt, N. et al. 2009. Human dendritic cells induce the differentiation of interleukin-21-producing T follicular helper-like cells through interleukin-12. Immunity 31: 158–169.

17. Schmitt, N. et al. 2013. IL-12 receptor β1 deficiency alters in vivo T follicular helper cell response in humans. Blood In press.

18. Saraiva, M. & A. O'Garra. The regulation of IL-10 production by immune cells. Nat. Rev. Immunol. 10: 170–181.

19. Hashimoto, D., J. Miller & M. Merad. 2011. Dendritic cell and macrophage heterogeneity in vivo. Immunity 35: 323–335.

20. Steinbrink, K. et al. 1999. Interleukin-10-treated human dendritic cells induce a melanoma-antigen-specific anergy in CD8(+) T cells resulting in a failure to lyse tumor cells. Blood 93: 1634–1642.

21. Li, M.O. & R.A. Flavell. 2008. Contextual regulation of inflammation: a duet by transforming growth factor-beta and interleukin-10. *Immunity* **28:** 468–476.

22. Tinoco, R. *et al.* 2009. Cell-intrinsic transforming growth factor-beta signaling mediates virus-specific CD8+ T cell deletion and viral persistence in vivo. *Immunity* **31:** 145–157.

23. Castro, A.G. *et al.* 2000. Anti-interleukin 10 receptor monoclonal antibody is an adjuvant for T helper cell type 1 responses to soluble antigen only in the presence of lipopolysaccharide. *J. Exp. Med.* **192:** 1529–1534.

24. Gorelik, L. & R.A. Flavell. 2002. Transforming growth factor-beta in T-cell biology. *Nat. Rev. Immunol.* **2:** 46–53.

25. Wrzesinski, S.H., Y.Y. Wan & R.A. Flavell. 2007. Transforming growth factor-beta and the immune response: implications for anticancer therapy. *Clin. Cancer Res.* **13:** 5262–5270.

26. Klebanoff, C.A. *et al.* 2004. IL-15 enhances the in vivo antitumor activity of tumor-reactive CD8+ T cells. *Proc. Natl. Acad. Sci. USA* **101:** 1969–1974.

27. Morris, J.C. *et al.* 2006. Preclinical and phase I clinical trial of blockade of IL-15 using Mikbeta1 monoclonal antibody in T cell large granular lymphocyte leukemia. *Proc. Natl. Acad. Sci. USA* **103:** 401–406.

28. Aspord, C. *et al.* 2007. Breast cancer instructs dendritic cells to prime interleukin 13-secreting CD4+ T cells that facilitate tumor development. *J. Exp. Med.* **204:** 1037–1047.

29. De Monte, L. *et al.* 2011. Intratumor T helper type 2 cell infiltrate correlates with cancer-associated fibroblast thymic stromal lymphopoietin production and reduced survival in pancreatic cancer. *J. Exp. Med.* **208:** 469–478.

30. Thomachot, M.C. *et al.* 2004. Breast carcinoma cells promote the differentiation of CD34+ progenitors towards 2 different subpopulations of dendritic cells with CD1a (high) CD86 (-) Langerin- and CD1a (+) CD86 (+) Langerin + phenotypes. *Int. J. Cancer* **110:** 710–720.

31. Vukmanovic-Stejic, M. *et al.* 2000. Human Tc1 and Tc2/Tc0 CD8 T-cell clones display distinct cell surface and functional phenotypes. *Blood* **95:** 231–240.

32. Maggi, E. *et al.* 1994. Th2-like CD8+ T cells showing B cell helper function and reduced cytolytic activity in human immunodeficiency virus type 1 infection. *J. Exp. Med.* **180:** 489–495.

33. Manetti, R. *et al.* 1994. CD30 expression by CD8+ T cells producing type 2 helper cytokines. Evidence for large numbers of CD8+ CD30+ T cell clones in human immunodeficiency virus infection. *J. Exp. Med.* **180:** 2407–2411.

34. Colonna, M. *et al.* 1998. Human myelomonocytic cells express an inhibitory receptor for classical and nonclassical MHC class I molecules. *J. Immunol.* **160:** 3096–3100.

35. Endo, S. *et al.* 2008. Regulation of cytotoxic T lymphocyte triggering by PIR-B on dendritic cells. *Proc. Natl. Acad. Sci. USA* **105:** 14515–14520.

36. Shiroishi, M. *et al.* 2003. Human inhibitory receptors Ig-like transcript 2 (ILT2) and ILT4 compete with CD8 for MHC class I binding and bind preferentially to HLA-G. *Proc. Natl. Acad. Sci. USA* **100:** 8856–8861.

37. Chang, C.C. *et al.* 2002. Tolerization of dendritic cells by T(S) cells: the crucial role of inhibitory receptors ILT3 and ILT4. *Nat. Immunol.* **3:** 237–243.

38. Ma, G. *et al.* 2011. Paired immunoglobin-like receptor-B regulates the suppressive function and fate of Myeloid-derived suppressor cells. *Immunity* **34:** 385–395.

39. Salgame, P. *et al.* 1991. Differing lymphokine profiles of functional subsets of human CD4 and CD8 T cell clones. *Science* **254:** 279–282.

40. Minkis, K. *et al.* 2008. Type 2 Bias of T cells expanded from the blood of melanoma patients switched to type 1 by IL-12p70 mRNA-transfected dendritic cells. *Cancer Res.* **68:** 9441–9450.

41. Roberts, W.K. *et al.* 2009. Patients with lung cancer and paraneoplastic Hu syndrome harbor HuD-specific type 2 CD8+ T cells. *J. Clin. Invest.* **119:** 2042–2051.

42. Sheu, B.C. *et al.* 2001. Predominant Th2/Tc2 polarity of tumor-infiltrating lymphocytes in human cervical cancer. *J. Immunol.* **167:** 2972–2978.

43. Maggi, E. *et al.* 1997. Functional characterization and modulation of cytokine production by CD8+ T cells from human immunodeficiency virus-infected individuals. *Blood* **89:** 3672–3681.

44. Nazaruk, R.A. *et al.* 1998. Functional diversity of the CD8(+) T-cell response to Epstein-Barr virus (EBV): implications for the pathogenesis of EBV-associated lymphoproliferative disorders. *Blood* **91:** 3875–3883.

45. Hermann, P. *et al.* 1995. CD40 ligand-positive CD8+ T cell clones allow B cell growth and differentiation. *Eur. J. Immunol.* **25:** 2972–2977.

46. Chu, C.C. *et al.* 2012. Resident CD141 (BDCA3)+ dendritic cells in human skin produce IL-10 and induce regulatory T cells that suppress skin inflammation. *J. Exp. Med.* **209:** 935–945.

47. Beck, S. & B.G. Barrell. 1988. Human cytomegalovirus encodes a glycoprotein homologous to MHC class-I antigens. *Nature* **331:** 269–272.

48. Robbins, S.H. *et al.* 2008. Novel insights into the relationships between dendritic cell subsets in human and mouse revealed by genome-wide expression profiling. *Genome Biol.* **9:** R17.

49. Jongbloed, S.L. *et al.* 2010. Human CD141+ (BDCA-3)+ dendritic cells (DCs) represent a unique myeloid DC subset that cross-presents necrotic cell antigens. *J. Exp. Med.* **207:** 1247–1260.

50. Bachem, A. *et al.* 2010. Superior antigen cross-presentation and XCR1 expression define human CD11c+ CD141+ cells as homologues of mouse CD8+ dendritic cells. *J. Exp. Med.* **207:** 1273–1281.

51. Crozat, K. *et al.* 2010. The XC chemokine receptor 1 is a conserved selective marker of mammalian cells homologous to mouse CD8alpha+ dendritic cells. *J. Exp. Med.* **207:** 1283–1292.

52. Poulin, L.F. *et al.* 2010. Characterization of human DNGR-1+ BDCA3+ leukocytes as putative equivalents of mouse CD8alpha+ dendritic cells. *J. Exp. Med.* **207:** 1261–1271.

53. Caminschi, I. *et al.* 2008. The dendritic cell subtype-restricted C-type lectin Clec9A is a target for vaccine enhancement. *Blood* **112:** 3264–3273.

54. de Sancho, D. & A. Rey. 2008. Energy minimizations with a combination of two knowledge-based potentials for protein folding. *J. Comput. Chem.* **29:** 1684–1692.

55. Joffre, O.P. *et al.* 2012. Cross-presentation by dendritic cells. *Nat. Rev. Immunol.* **12:** 557–569.

56. Segura, E. *et al.* 2012. Characterization of resident and migratory dendritic cells in human lymph nodes. *J. Exp. Med.* **209:** 653–660.

57. Bonifaz, L. *et al.* 2002. Efficient targeting of protein antigen to the dendritic cell receptor DEC-205 in the steady state leads to antigen presentation on major histocompatibility complex class I products and peripheral CD8[+] T cell tolerance. *J. Exp. Med.* **196:** 1627–1638.

58. Bozzacco, L. *et al.* 2007. DEC-205 receptor on dendritic cells mediates presentation of HIV gag protein to CD8[+] T cells in a spectrum of human MHC I haplotypes. *Proc. Natl. Acad. Sci. USA* **104:** 1289–1294.

59. Dudziak, D. *et al.* 2007. Differential antigen processing by dendritic cell subsets in vivo. *Science* **315:** 107–111.

60. Klechevsky, E. *et al.* 2010. Cross-priming CD8[+] T cells by targeting antigens to human dendritic cells through DCIR. *Blood* **116:** 1685–1697.

61. Idoyaga, J. *et al.* 2009. Antibody to Langerin/CD207 localizes large numbers of CD8alpha[+] dendritic cells to the marginal zone of mouse spleen. *Proc. Natl. Acad. Sci. USA* **106:** 1524–1529.

62. Sancho, D. *et al.* 2008. Tumor therapy in mice via antigen targeting to a novel, DC-restricted C-type lectin. *J. Clin. Invest.* **118:** 2098–2110.

63. Hodi, F.S. *et al.* 2010. Improved survival with ipilimumab in patients with metastatic melanoma. *N. Engl. J. Med.* **363:** 711–723.

Ann. N.Y. Acad. Sci. ISSN 0077-8923

ANNALS OF THE NEW YORK ACADEMY OF SCIENCES

Issue: *The Renaissance of Cancer Immunotherapy*

Dendritic cell immunotherapy

Rachel Lubong Sabado and Nina Bhardwaj

NYU Langone Medical Center Cancer Institute, New York University School of Medicine, New York, New York

Address for correspondence: Nina Bhardwaj, Tumor Vaccine Program, NYU Langone Medical Center Cancer Institute, New York University School of Medicine, 522 First Avenue, SRB 1303, New York, NY 10016. Nina.Bhardwaj@nyumc.org

The U.S. Food and Drug Administration's approval of the first cell-based immunotherapy has rejuvenated interest in the field. Early clinical trials have established the ability of dendritic cell (DC) immunotherapy to exploit a patient's own immune system to induce antitumor immune responses. However, suboptimal conditions for generating potent immunostimulatory DCs, in addition to the suppression mediated by the tumor microenvironment, have contributed to limited clinical success *in vivo*. Therefore, combining DC vaccines with new approaches that enhance immunogenicity and overcome the regulatory mechanisms underlying peripheral tolerance may be key to achieving effective, durable, antitumor immune responses that translate to better clinical outcomes.

Keywords: dendritic cells; immunotherapy; cancer; vaccine

Introduction

Dendritic cells (DCs) are the most potent antigen-presenting cells (APC), capable of activating both naive and memory immune responses. Clinical trials of antigen-pulsed DCs conducted in patients in various tumor settings have demonstrated that antigen-loaded DC vaccines are safe and promising therapeutic approaches for tumors. However, their clinical efficacy remains to be established.

Dendritic cell biology

DCs have a superior capacity for acquiring and processing antigens for presentation to T cells, and express high levels of costimulatory/coinhibitory molecules that determine immune activation or anergy.[1] The Nobel Prize in Medicine or Physiology was awarded to Ralph Steinman in 2011 for discovering DCs almost 40 years ago.

Myeloid (mDC) and plasmacytoid (pDC) are the two major types of DCs. mDCs are found in peripheral tissues, lymphoid organs, and in the blood, and secrete large amounts of interleukin-12 (IL-12) upon activation, driving immune responses against pathogenic organisms or suppressing neoplastic cell growth.[2,3] pDCs are primarily found in the blood and lymphoid organs and can produce up to 1000-fold more type I IFNs in response to viral infections than other cell types.[4] Additionally, pDCs may play a dual role in immune responses against tumors.[5] Although pDCs can activate melanoma-specific CD8+ T cell responses,[6] pDCs may also inhibit antitumor immune responses. pDCs with diminished capacity to produce IFN-α, which is critical for preventing the establishment of tumors through enhancement of innate and adaptive immune responses,[7] have been found in many tumors.[6,8] Furthermore, pDCs expressing indoleamine 2,3 dioxygenase (IDO), which is responsible for the degradation of tryptophan, an amino acid essential for T cell proliferation and implicated in the generation of regulatory T cells, have also been located in tumor-draining lymph nodes.[9–12]

DCs take up antigens through phagocytosis, macropinocytosis, or endocytosis using Fc receptors (Fcγ receptor types I (CD64) and II (CD32)), integrins ($\alpha_v\beta_3$ or $\alpha_v\beta_5$), C-type lectins (mannose receptor, DEC205), apoptotic cell receptors, and scavenger receptors. Protein antigens are processed into peptides that are loaded on MHC molecules for presentation to T cells. DCs can also process antigens via cross-presentation. Although the precise mechanism of cross-presentation remains controversial, the ability of DCs to utilize this process to activate CD8+ T cells has been well established in many cases.[1,13,14] DCs can process lipid antigens and then

doi: 10.1111/nyas.12125

present on CD1d molecules to activate natural killer T (NKT) cells, and DCs can recognize and uptake antigens containing carbohydrate structures via C-type lectin receptors (CLR), (i.e., MMR, DEC-205, and DC-SIGN). CLRs can function as endocytic receptors to internalize antigens for antigen processing and presentation;[15,16] however, some of these C-type lectin receptors (i.e., MICL, DICR) may be inhibitory.[17]

Maturation of DCs is characterized by reduced phagocytic capacity, enhanced processing and presentation, enhanced migration to lymphoid tissues, and increased stimulation of B and T cells. Maturation is induced by microbial products through activation of pattern recognition receptors (PRR) such as Toll-like receptors (TLRs),[18] or via activation of endogenous sensors such as RIG-I,[19] members of the inflammasome,[20] or inflammatory molecules (TNF-α, IL-1, IL-6, and IFN-α) produced by the cells of the immune system or by damaged tissues.[21] Maturation is accompanied by increased expression of chemokine receptors, adhesion molecules, and costimulatory molecules that are important for migration to lymphoid tissues and for optimal activation of immune responses. Cytokines produced during this process influence immune responses generated by differentiating subtypes of CD4$^+$ T cells such as T helper 1 (Th1), Th2, Th17, and regulatory T cells. Besides T cells, DCs activate naive and memory B cells,[22] natural killer (NK) cells (via IL-12, IL-15, and type I IFNs),[23] and NKT cells through antigen presentation on CD1 molecules.[24] Thus, DCs can qualitatively and quantitatively orchestrate immune responses.

In addition to immunity, DCs mediate peripheral tolerance and prevent autoimmunity.[25,26] Immature DCs do not activate T cells because they express low levels of MHC and costimulatory molecules. DCs may also induce the expression of IDO, which drives T cells to undergo cell cycle arrest or apoptosis. Tryptophan metabolites produced by DCs also exert direct cytotoxic effects on T cells.[27,28] DCs can induce the differentiation of regulatory T cells,[29,30] which can infiltrate several tumors[31,32] and exert their effects through TGF-β, IL-10, and CTLA-4, among other mechanisms, to inhibit proliferating T cells.[26,33] DCs can also mediate tolerance to self-antigens through the uptake of apoptotic cells via receptors, including LOX-1, CD36, $\alpha_v\beta_3$, $\alpha_v\beta_5$, and the complement receptors (CRs) CR3 and CR4.

Ligation of CR3 by apoptotic cells on DCs leads to impaired maturation in response to stimulation with LPS and impaired priming and activation of memory T cell responses.[34] Furthermore, binding of apoptotic microparticles to CD44 induced inhibition of DCs.[35] Gut mucosa CD103$^+$ DCs have an enhanced ability to metabolize vitamin A, and generate retinoic acid, which drives the differentiation of gut-homing regulatory T cells.[36]

Dendritic cells for tumor immunotherapy

Insights into the role of the immune system in eliminating tumors have come from reports of spontaneous regression of primary and metastatic melanoma;[37] the existence of immunogenic tumor-associated or specific antigens;[38] the significantly higher risk of tumor development in knockout mice lacking components of the IFN-γ signaling pathways, perforin, or recombination activating gene 1/2 (RAG1/2);[39] and the adoptive transfer of tumor-infiltrating lymphocytes (TILs) that induce objective regression of tumors in melanoma patients.[38] Furthermore, T cell infiltration of tumor sites has been associated with longer disease-free survival and/or overall survival in various tumor settings.[40] On the basis of these findings, investigators hypothesize that DCs would serve as ideal tools for boosting endogenous antitumor responses that may lead to the effective eradication of tumors. DCs can be loaded with tumor antigens and injected back into patients where they would traffic into lymphoid tissues and activate antigen-specific T cells that could kill the tumor (Fig. 1). In support of this, early clinical trials using *ex vivo*–generated DCs pulsed with tumor antigens demonstrated that immune responses could indeed be induced, thus fueling further studies, summarized below, designed to manipulate DCs to enhance immune responses *in vivo*.

Preparation
The methods for generating DCs used in clinical trials include differentiation from monocyte precursors, CD34$^+$ hematopoietic precursors, and *in vivo* expansion of circulating DCs. Although a comparison of the transcriptional profile of DCs generated by various methods provides evidence of fundamental differences of their functionality *in vivo*,[41] no direct comparison of the different methods of DC generation has been tested in clinical trials. Despite this, DCs derived using these different

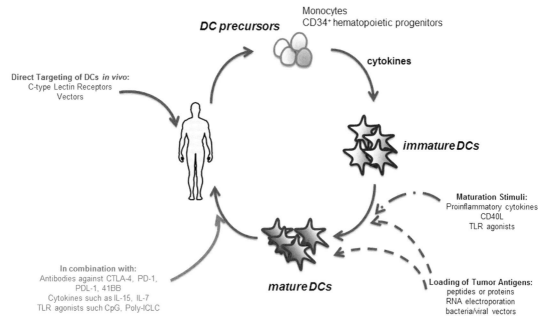

Figure 1. DC immunotherapy. DC precursors (monocytes or CD34$^+$ hematopoietic progenitor cells) are isolated from patients from large blood draws or leukapheresis collections. Immature DCs are differentiated from monocytes using GM-CSF and IL-4 and CD34$^+$ hematopoietic cells using GM-CSF, FLt3L, and TNF-α for one or more weeks. The addition of proinflammatory cytokines, CD40L, or TLR agonists to the immature DCs induces the maturation of DCs in 1–2 days. Tumor antigens in the form of proteins or peptides are either loaded with the addition of maturation stimuli or after DCs are matured. Once matured and loaded with tumor antigens, DCs can be frozen in aliquots and thawed just before injection or can be injected fresh to the patient. To further enhance its function *in vivo*, DCs can be injected in combination with antibodies (CTLA-4, PD-1, PDL-1, 41BB), cytokines (IL-15, IL-7, IL-12), or TLR agonists (CpG, poly-I:C). Alternatively, *in vivo* DCs can be activated by direct targeting using DC-specific receptors and vectors that carry antigens and maturation stimuli or using TLR agonists coinjected with antigens. The injected/activated DCs then migrate to lymphoid tissues to activate antigen-specific CD4$^+$ and CD8$^+$ T cells. Upon activation, antigen-specific CD4$^+$ and CD8$^+$ T cells traffic out of the lymphoid tissues and inhibit the growth of tumors.

methods have stimulated antigen-specific T cell responses in both preclinical and clinical studies.

The most common approach involves the differentiation of DCs from peripheral blood mononuclear cells (PBMC) obtained from whole blood or leukapheresis, called monocyte-derived DC (MDDC). CD14$^+$ monocytes are selected from PBMCs by plastic adherence or positive selection using immunomagnetic beads.[42–46] These monocytes are induced to differentiate into immature CD14$^-$ CD83$^-$ DCs in culture for several days in the presence of IL-4 and GM-CSF, and stimulated to mature by culturing for an additional 1–2 days in the presence of a maturation stimulus.

DCs are also propagated from CD34$^+$ precursors that are mobilized from the bone marrow by treatment of patients with G-CSF before harvesting by leukapheresis.[47] The harvested cells are further expanded *in vitro* for one week or more in the presence of GM-CSF, Flt3L, and TNF-α, producing a mixture of MDDCs, DCs that are phenotypically similar to epidermal Langerhans cells (LC), and a large proportion of myeloid cells at different stages of differentiation. Interestingly, the LCs, not the DCs, may be the cell type from this mixture that is responsible for stimulating T cell responses.[48] However, comparison of melanoma peptide-loaded LCs and MDDCs revealed that although LCs were more potent stimulators of antigen-specific T cell responses than MDDCs, MDDCs supplemented with IL-15 stimulated significantly more antigen-specific effector memory T cells.[49]

Administration of growth factors such as Flt3L induces the *in vivo* expansion of circulating DCs.[50] Daily administration of Flt3L for 10 days led to a 48-fold expansion of mDCs and 13-fold expansion of pDCs. Expanded DC subsets upregulated maturation markers, produced cytokines upon stimulation, and stimulated T cell responses. However, expanded DC subsets elicited distinct cytokine profiles in the stimulated $CD4^+$ T cells, with the expanded pDCs inducing higher levels of IL-10.[51] Administration of Flt3L may also expand NK cells.[52] Dendreon's Provenge® (sipuleucel-T), a vaccine using DC-enriched peripheral blood, was the first FDA-approved cell-based therapy for the treatment of hormone-refractory prostate cancer.[53] In addition to DCs, Provenge also contains B cells, monocytes, and NK cells that are cultured *ex vivo* with a recombinant fusion protein containing prostatic acid phosphatase (PAP) and GM-CSF, before being administered back into patients within 48 hours of the leukapheresis collection.[54]

Maturation

Maturation of DCs is critical, as mature DCs have enhanced expression of costimulatory molecules, produce cytokines and chemokines necessary for the efficient activation of T cell responses,[1] and exhibit enhanced migration to lymphoid tissues.[55] Furthermore, immature DCs fail to induce antigen-specific responses[56] and may induce the differentiation of regulatory T cells.[26,57] Peptide-loaded mature DCs, not immature DCs, induced antigen-specific T cell responses in patients with metastatic melanoma.[58]

The majority of clinical trials using DCs have used a cocktail of proinflammatory cytokines to mature the DCs.[59] This cocktail of cytokines consisting of TNF-α, IL-1β, IL-6, and PGE_2 has been demonstrated to induce the upregulation of MHC class I and II, CD40, CD80, CD86, and CCR7 after 2 days of culture, but no IL-12p70.[59] Despite the lack of IL-12p70 production, when compared to other DC maturation stimuli (CD40L trimer, poly I:C, and LPS), the cytokine cocktail induced the most uniform upregulation of DC maturation markers, the highest yields and recovery, stimulated the highest levels of allogeneic T cell proliferation and cytokine production, and induced the priming of Th1 responses.[59] Nonetheless, studies indicate that the presence of PGE_2 in the cocktail may induce differentiation of regulatory T cells and Th2 responses,[60] IDO expression,[61] deficiency in IL-12p70 production,[62] and inhibit migration through induction of tissue inhibitors of metalloproteinases (TIMP).[63] Interestingly, PGE_2 has also been shown to be critical for the migration of DCs into lymphoid tissues through upregulation of CCR7[64] and the enhancing of T cell proliferation through induction of OX40L, CD70, and 4–1BBL in DCs.[65] Therefore, the cytokine cocktail may be playing a dual role in the development of antitumor responses.

Others have explored the use of alternative methods of maturing DCs. CD40 ligand (CD40L) has been used to mature DCs for vaccination in clinical trials.[43] CD40L, expressed primarily by activated T cells and B cells, is a principal component of $CD4^+$ T cell help that binds to CD40 on DCs and induces DC maturation. Because TLR activation differentially stimulates systemic and local innate immune responses *in vivo*,[66] the use of TLR agonists has also been explored. TLR activation on DCs induces maturation, upregulation of costimulatory molecules, and production of cytokines and chemokines.[67] Furthermore, simultaneous triggering of different TLRs on DCs mediate synergistic effects on DC function, resulting in the production of supramolecular levels of IL-12.[68,69] Thus, TLR agonists have the potential to induce optimal DCs for stimulating effective immune responses and conditioning the environment *in vivo* to favor the development of immune responses. A novel cytokine cocktail consisting of TNF-α, IL-1β, polyinosinic:polycytidylic acid (Poly-ICLC), IFN-α, and IFN-γ induces the maturation of DCs called α type 1-polarized DCs (αDC1s). These αDC1s produced high levels of IL-12p70, migrated in response to CCR7 ligands, and induced CTL responses against tumor-associated antigens (TAAs).[70,71] Administration of αDC1s in patients with high-grade glioma was safe and immunogenic, and resulted in progression-free status lasting at least 12 months in 9 of 22 patients.[72] Alternatively, others have used *in situ* maturation strategies via preconditioning of injection sites with cytokines,[73] TLR agonists,[74] or injection of DCs that are partially matured,[75] which have resulted in induction of immune responses.

Antigen loading

The method of delivery for antigens is important in determining the activation of $CD4^+$ and/or $CD8^+$ T cells. DCs are typically loaded through incubation with peptides, proteins, or actual irradiated tumor cells.[46] Peptides are loaded directly onto MHC class molecules on the surface of the DCs, whereas the use of proteins and tumor cells requires processing into peptides before loading on MHC molecules. Once loaded with antigens, the DCs are frozen in aliquots and thawed as needed for the vaccinations.[46]

There are now a number of TAAs for T cells from a variety of tumors that can be exploited for immunotherapy. Short synthetic peptides (8–15 aa) that correspond to defined epitopes within these TAAs have been used in clinical trials. However, use of these short peptides necessitates the knowledge of patient haplotypes and the defined epitopes that would bind these specific haplotypes. More recently, synthetic long peptides (SLP) that are 28–35 aa long have been used.[76] Because of their length, SLPs are unable to bind directly to MHC molecules. SLPs are preferentially taken up, processed, and presented by DCs through cross-presentation,[77] leading to activation of both CD4[+] and CD8[+] T cell responses. Studies using SLPs covering the entire length of HPV-16 E6 and E7 protein in patients with advanced HPV-16[+] cervical cancer showed that the vaccine was safe and immunogenic.[78,79] In another study, 79% of patients vaccinated with the HPV-16 SLP with Montanide ISA-51 had objective responses after 12 months with no evidence of virus at original lesions in five patients.[80] On the basis of the success of these studies, vaccine formulations using SLPs have been further explored in cervical,[81] ovarian,[82,83] and colorectal cancer,[84,85] and HIV.[86]

DCs loaded with proteins[87] and autologous or allogeneic tumors/tumor cell lines[43,88–91] or lysates[92,93] have also been used in numerous cancers. Multiple epitopes that are presented on different haplotypes have the potential to induce immune responses to a wide spectrum of antigens, while the requirement for processing results in prolonged antigen presentation.[94] Furthermore, studies using proteins or tumor cells have reported the induction of CD8[+] T cell responses, indicating the activation of cross-presentation pathways.

Bacteria such as *Mycobacterium bovis*, *Listeria monocytogenes*, *Salmonella*, and *Shigella*, and viruses such as Canarypox, Newcastle disease, vaccinia, Sindbis, yellow fever, human papillomavirus, adenovirus, adeno-associated virus, and lentiviruses have been explored for use as vectors.[42,95–100] Genes encoding TAAs are inserted into the vector, while genes encoding virulence or replication factors are deleted. These vectors have the ability to elicit natural immune responses against the vector of choice, thereby enhancing the immunogenicity of TAAs. Some vectors may also induce the matura-tion of DCs, thus bypassing the need for a separate maturation stimulus. Infecting DCs with a killed, but metabolically active (KBMA) *Listeria monocytogenes* encoding an epitope of MelanA/Mart-1 induced maturation of the DCs, priming of Mart-1–specific CD8[+] T cells, and lysis of patient-derived melanoma cells *in vitro*. Furthermore, KBMA efficiently targeted APCs *in vivo* to induce protective antitumor responses in a mouse tumor model.[101] However, preexisting immunity against the vector may limit its ability to induce immune responses *in vivo*.

Lentivirus-based vectors have several properties that offer distinct advantages over vectors currently used in clinical trials.[102,103] Although lentivirus-based vectors are typically less immunogenic, they have the potential to trigger endosomal or cytoplasmic sensors (e.g., TLRs, RIG-I, and PKR) to activate the innate immune system. Lentivirus-based vectors have the additional capacity to transduce quiescent and nondividing cells such as MDDCs, which are usually propagated from quiescent CD14[+] or CD34[+] progenitors.[104–107] Lentivirus-based vectors have induced strong antitumor CD8[+] T cell responses, primed tumor-specific T cell responses *in vitro*,[108] and inhibited the growth of preexisting tumors in mouse models.[109,110] Additionally, lentiviral-based vectors have the potential for use as a vehicle for direct therapeutic vaccination. The *in vivo* use of the lentiviral vector pseudotyped with glycoprotein specific for DC-SIGN from Sindbis virus resulted in the efficient transduction and maturation of DCs and the activation of immune responses.[111] Therefore, with improved biosafety, these vectors can deliver antigens to DCs both *in vitro* and *in vivo* and induce effective tumor-specific immune responses.

DCs can be transfected directly with RNA without the use of vectors. DCs loaded with mRNA encoding TAAs have been demonstrated to induce potent tumor antigen-specific T cell responses.[112–115] Although transfection of DCs with mRNA can be accomplished with the use of a cationic lipid (i.e., DOTAP) or mRNA alone, electroporation has been demonstrated to be the most efficient method to introduce mRNA into DCs by temporarily increasing permeability.[116] Electroporation of DCs has been successfully used in preclinical[117–119] and clinical[120] studies for tumor immunotherapy. Electroporation of autologous DCs with RNA encoding CD40L and

HIV antigens was demonstrated to be safe and to induce HIV-specific immune responses.[121]

Direct targeting of antigens to *in vivo* DCs to induce tumor-specific immune responses[122,123] is a novel strategy that bypasses the expensive and labor-intensive *ex vivo* DC generation process. This strategy allows for vaccines to be produced on a larger scale and, more importantly, stimulates the activation of natural DC subsets at multiple sites *in vivo*. Early approaches of targeting *in vivo* DCs involved engineering irradiated tumor cells to secrete GM-CSF[124,125] to stimulate the recruitment and enhance the function of APCs. However, prolonged GM-CSF production in the tumor microenvironment has been associated with disease progression in some experimental models and in a phase III trial in patients with hormone therapy–refractory prostate cancer,[125] likely due to recruitment of myeloid suppressor cells or differentiation of myeloid precursors into immature tolerogenic dendritic cells.[126,127] In contrast, a clinical trial in pancreatic adenocarcinoma showed that vaccination with lethally irradiated allogeneic GM-CSF–secreting tumor vaccine induced antigen-specific CD8$^+$ T cells that correlated with prolonged disease-free survival in HLA-matched patients[128] and have been supported in animal models of pancreatic cancer.[129]

Newer approaches involve the targeting of DCs using DC-specific molecules such as Fc receptors, CD40, and C-type lectin receptors (CLR). CLRs are the most attractive targets, as different DC subsets are known to express different CLRs that are involved in the recognition and capture of many glycosylated antigens.[130] Studies targeting antigens to CLRs with a DC-activating stimulus resulted in the effective generation of T cell responses[131–133] and enhancement of antibody responses.[134] Recent studies using DEC205-targeting antibodies have successfully induced immune responses to both cancer[135] and HIV.[136,137] Although the majority of these studies are performed in mice, human studies using DC-SIGN,[138] MR,[139] and DEC205[140] have demonstrated successful induction of tumor-specific T cell responses.

Administration

The effective migration of DC vaccines is critical to the success of the vaccines. Although DC vaccines have been administered using various routes (intradermally, subcutaneously, intravenously, or intra-

tumorally), the optimal route of administration for DC vaccines has yet to be established. Tracking of 111-indium–labeled MDDC loaded with melanoma peptides and administered intradermally revealed that large numbers of injected DCs remained at the injection site, lost viability, and cleared within 48 hours. More importantly, <5% of DC vaccines reached the draining lymph nodes.[141] Migration did not improve with intratumoral administration, as DCs remained at the injection sites and none were detected in the draining lymph nodes.[142,143]

The need to improve the migration of injected DCs to lymphoid tissues is critical for stimulating effective immune responses. Newer strategies include administration of DC vaccines via multiple routes (i.e., intradermally and intravenously) to induce a systemic response or administration directly to the lymph nodes (intranodally). Intranodally administered MDDC loaded with melanoma peptides redistributed to multiple lymph nodes within 30 minutes of injection. However, despite direct delivery of DCs into the lymph nodes, immunologic responses elicited were comparable[141] or not better[143] than intradermally administered DC vaccine. Reducing the number of cells injected improved migration of DCs[144] as well as injection of immature DC into skin preconditioned with the TLR7 agonist imiquimod.[75] Interestingly, a mouse model revealed that DC vaccines are not responsible for activating T cells. DC vaccines act as vehicles for transferring antigens to endogenous APCs that are directly responsible for activating T cell responses.[145] Thus, further studies are required to enhance the migration of DC vaccines in order to directly or indirectly induce immune responses.

Improving DC immunotherapy

Overall, clinical trials have demonstrated the feasibility and safety of DC vaccines. Observed side effects were relatively mild and transient and include fever, injection site reactions, adenopathy, and fatigue. Nonetheless, despite the induction of tumor-specific T cell responses in many patients and occasional complete tumor regressions, DC vaccines have not translated into meaningful therapeutic responses.

The lack of consensus on the optimal DC for immunotherapeutic use may be a major contributing factor to the limited success for DC vaccines. As described above, DCs used in clinical trials were derived using different methods and administered using various routes. Although these studies have provided promising results from phase I and II trials, immune responses that correlate with clinical responses have failed to translate in large phase III trials.[146,147] The tumor microenvironment employs mechanisms that include loss of tumor antigen expression, alteration of MHC molecules, lack of costimulation, expression of inhibitory ligands, induction of regulatory T cells, expression of IDO, and/or production of immunosuppressive cytokines[28,148–151] that may inhibit the capacity of DC vaccines to induce immune responses against the tumor. Therefore, studies focused on optimizing DC preparation in combination with approaches that overcome immune evasive mechanisms by the tumor microenvironment will likely improve efficacies of DC vaccines *in vivo*. Newer strategies addressing these issues are now being tested in clinical trials.

Targeting immune checkpoint molecules has been shown to enhance immune responses.[152,153] Antibodies blocking the interaction of DCs with PD-1 on activated T cells have been shown to enhance tumor-specific immune responses *in vitro*.[154–156] The phase I studies of the antibody against PD-1 demonstrated safety in patients and increased the percentage of peripheral blood CD4[+] lymphocytes in patients with advanced hematologic malignancies[157] and resulted in one complete and two partial remissions in patients with colorectal cancer, melanoma, and renal cell carcinoma and significant tumor regressions in two additional patients with melanoma and non-small-cell lung cancer.[158] Additionally, a recent study reported that although 18% of patients had grade 3 or 4 adverse events, 18% of non-small-cell lung cancer, 28% of melanoma, and 27% of renal-cell cancer patients who received anti-PD-1 had durable clinical responses.[159] Similarly, a study using anti-PDL-1 reported durable clinical responses and prolonged disease stabilization along with grade 3 or 4 adverse events.[160] Clinical trials of two CTLA-4 blocking antibodies, ipilimumab and tremelimumab, in melanoma showed promising clinical responses.[161] Ipilimumab (Yervoy[TM]) has since been approved by the FDA for the treatment of unresectable or metastatic melanoma, based on improved overall survival in treated patients.[162] In addition, anti-CTLA-4 blocking antibodies are currently under investigation in other malignancies such as prostate cancer, renal cell carcinoma, and non-Hodgkin's lymphoma.[163] The 4-1BB/CD137 receptor pair is expressed by activated T cells and is implicated in the survival of activated and memory CD8[+] T cells.[164] Antibody against 4-1BB enhanced rejection of large tumors by promoting survival of CD8[+] T cells,[165] likely mediated through DCs.[166] Furthermore, combination with anti-CTLA-4 enhanced tumor-specific immunity while reducing autoimmune responses.[167] In an open-label phase I–II study, administration of anti-4-1BB to patients with locally advanced or metastatic solid tumors resulted in partial remissions and stable disease. However, other clinical studies using anti-41BB were terminated due to toxicity.[168] DCs expressing CD40 engage its cognate ligand CD40L on CD4[+] T cells, leading to enhancement of expression of costimulatory molecules and cytokines and more efficient cross-presentation by DCs.[169] The use of CD40 agonists has also been explored.[170] CD40 agonist antibody in combination with gemcitabine chemotherapy was tested in a clinical trial of patients with pancreatic ductal adenocarcinoma.[171] The investigators showed that it was the CD40-activated macrophages, not T cells or chemotherapy, that mediated the destruction of the tumor, thereby highlighting the importance of targeting cells other than T cells for immunotherapy.

Cytokines have been shown to enhance T cell survival and function. IL-15 promotes the induction of longer-lived and higher-avidity CD8[+] T cells[172] with the capacity to effectively kill tumor cells[173] and reverse T cell anergy.[174] Furthermore, IL-15 administration enhances the differentiation and proliferation of NK cells, differentiation and antibody production of B cells,[175] and in combination with IL-21 further enhances T cell function.[176] A clinical trial using IL-15 in metastatic malignant melanoma and renal cell cancer is underway and should provide more information on its effectiveness *in vivo*.[177] IL-7 is required for T cell development and naive T cell survival in the periphery.[178] Phase I trials established that administration of IL-7 dramatically increases total CD4[+] and CD8[+] T cell populations without increasing regulatory T cell numbers.[179] IL-12, a critical cytokine for development of Th1 responses, can also be used to enhance immune responses. Transfection of DCs with a gene encoding IL-12 skewed Th2 responses from melanoma patients into Th1 responses.[180] Additionally, IL-12 has been shown to enhance NK cell cytotoxicity and IFN-γ production[181] and has led to high rates of T cell activation and generation of complement-fixing, tumor-lytic antibodies[182] within lymph nodes. Furthermore, administration of IL-12 fused to tumor-targeting antibody was safe and resulted in partial response and disease shrinkage in melanoma patients.[183] Targeting immunosuppressive cytokines such as IL-10 and TGF-β will likely enhance the vaccine's effectiveness. Combination therapy of TLR9 agonist CpG and IL-10R antibody enhanced the tumor-specific immune response and triggered *de novo* IL-12 production.[184] Furthermore, inhibition of TGF-β suppressed the proliferation of regulatory T cells and increased the number of tumor antigen-specific T cells;[185] the prolonged survival of DC-vaccinated melanoma patients correlated with the reduction of TGF-β-expressing T cells.[186]

Potentiation of immune responses through the use of TLR agonists is being actively pursued. Combining TLR7 agonist imiquimod[74] and TLR9 agonist CpG ODN[187] with tumor antigens for adjuvant therapy resulted in enhanced tumor antigen-specific immune responses. Topically applied imiquimod induced infiltration of mononuclear cells, including T cells, monocytes, NK cells, mDCs, and, to a lesser extent, pDCs, and resulted in the activation of humoral and cellular responses.[74] The TLR3 agonist poly I:C was shown to be superior to other TLR agonists (CpG, R848, LPS, Pam3cys, and Malp-2) in inducing CD4+ T cells.[188] Furthermore, the simultaneous triggering of multiple TLR agonists mediates synergistic effects.[68] Combinations of TLR agonists have induced rapid and sustained activation of DCs and enhanced CTL effector functions,[189] induced DCs to produce high levels of IL-12 and to migrate in response to CCR7 ligands,[69] and induced integrated immune responses.[190] Therefore, further studies exploring the uses of TLR agonists are likely to be beneficial.

Additional strategies for enhancing immune responses are under exploration. Nonspecific immunomodulators such as Montanide™, a water-in-oil emulsion similar to incomplete Freund's adjuvant, has been used in a number of clinical studies.[191,192] Although Montanide, in combination with TLR agonists, has been demonstrated to induce expansion of tumor antigen-specific CD8+ T cells

in melanoma patients,[193] intriguing data presented at the 2012 Cancer Research Institute Cancer Immunotherapy Symposium indicate that Montanide promotes a persistent, antigen-rich depot that leads to sequestering of vaccine-primed T cells instead of allowing these T cells to localize to tumors.[41] Targeting NKT cells may be another option, as dysfunctional NKT cells have been observed in several advanced malignancies.[194] In addition to its direct antitumor effects, DC-NKT crosstalk may further potentiate DC activation and IL-12 production. In a phase I study, α-GalCer–loaded mature DCs injected into patients with advanced cancer led to *in vivo* expansion and activation of NKT cells, and was associated with increases in serum levels of IL-12p40 and IP-10 and antigen-specific T cell responses.[195] Heterologous prime-boost immunizations may also improve efficacy of DC vaccines. Because the prime vaccine vector is different from the boost vaccine vector, the vaccine induces a more immunogenic response compared to a homologous prime boost. This has been demonstrated in cancer patients who have received different prime-and-boost vaccination protocols.[196,197] The use of standard chemotherapeutic agents in combination with DC vaccines may also enhance efficacy by enhancing antigen presentation of DCs *in vivo*[198,199] and by altering the phenotype of tumor cells and rendering them more susceptible to lysis by T cells.[200,201] Finally, taking advantage of the development of intravital two-photon imaging to track DC vaccines *in vivo* to gain new insights into their function and interaction with the rest of the immune system should provide additional strategies for optimization.[202]

Conclusion

Clinical studies using *ex vivo* DCs demonstrated that immune responses against TAAs can be induced, and in cases such as HIV, have yielded exciting results. Patients vaccinated with autologous MDDC pulsed with aldrithiol-2–inactivated autologous HIV-suppressed viral loads for at least a year positively correlated with HIV-specific CD4+ and CD8+ T cell responses.[203] In another study, HIV-1 patients were randomized to receive either autologous MDDC pulsed with autologous heat-inactivated whole HIV or unpulsed autologous MDDC. DC vaccination was safe and immunogenic, and control of viral replication following treatment interruption was associated with the vaccine.[204] However, the limited clinical responses in the majority of DC vaccine studies emphasize the need for further optimization of DC vaccine protocols. Our group demonstrates this in a recent unpublished study in melanoma patients. An emulsion of montanide and melanoma peptides was better, in terms of frequency and magnitude, at stimulating immune responses than *ex vivo* cytokine–matured DCs loaded with the same melanoma peptides (O'Neill *et al.*, submitted). Although immunotherapy with *ex vivo*–derived DCs may eventually give way to cheaper and less cumbersome preparations, the lessons learned from these studies have provided and continue to provide valuable new strategies for inducing antitumor immune responses *in vivo*. Altogether, these new strategies may be the keys to enhancing tumor immunity *in vivo* that can translate into meaningful clinical outcomes.

Conflicts of interest

Nina Bhardwaj is a coinventor on patents relating to DC manufacture.

References

1. Banchereau, J. *et al.* 2000. Immunobiology of dendritic cells. *Annu. Rev. Immunol.* **18:** 767–811.
2. Trinchieri, G. 2003. Interleukin-12 and the regulation of innate resistance and adaptive immunity. *Nat. Rev. Immunol.* **3:** 133–146.
3. Vignali, D.A. & V.K. Kuchroo. 2012. IL-12 family cytokines: immunological playmakers. *Nat. Immunol.* **13:** 722–728.
4. McKenna, K., A.S. Beignon & N. Bhardwaj. 2005. Plasmacytoid dendritic cells: linking innate and adaptive immunity. *J. Virol.* **79:** 17–27.
5. Tel, J. *et al.* 2012. Harnessing human plasmacytoid dendritic cells as professional APCs. *Cancer Immunol. Immunother.* **61:** 1279–1288.
6. Salio, M. *et al.* 2003. Plasmacytoid dendritic cells prime IFN-gamma-secreting melanoma-specific CD8 lymphocytes and are found in primary melanoma lesions. *Eur. J. Immunol.* **33:** 1052–1062.
7. Dunn, G. P. *et al.* 2005. A critical function for type I interferons in cancer immunoediting. *Nat. Immunol.* **6:** 722–729.
8. Hartmann, E. *et al.* 2003. Identification and functional analysis of tumor-infiltrating plasmacytoid dendritic cells in head and neck cancer. *Cancer Res.* **63:** 6478–6487.
9. Gerlini, G. *et al.* 2007. Plasmacytoid dendritic cells represent a major dendritic cell subset in sentinel lymph nodes of melanoma patients and accumulate in metastatic nodes. *Clin. Immunol.* **125:** 184–193.
10. Battaglia, A. *et al.* 2009. Metastatic tumour cells favour the generation of a tolerogenic milieu in tumour draining lymph node in patients with early cervical cancer. *Cancer Immunol. Immunother.* **58:** 1363–1373.
11. Sharma, M.D. *et al.* 2007. Plasmacytoid dendritic cells from mouse tumor-draining lymph nodes directly activate mature Tregs via indoleamine 2,3-dioxygenase. *J. Clin, Invest.* **117:** 2570–2582.
12. Munn, D.H. *et al.* 2004. Expression of indoleamine 2,3-dioxygenase by plasmacytoid dendritic cells in tumor-draining lymph nodes. *J. Clin. Invest.* **114:** 280–290.
13. Guermonprez, P. *et al.* 2002. Antigen presentation and T cell stimulation by dendritic cells. *Annu. Rev. Immunol.* **20:** 621–667.
14. Joffre, O.P. *et al.* 2012. Cross-presentation by dendritic cells. Nature reviews. *Immunology* **12:** 557–569.
15. Cambi, A., M. Koopman & C.G. Figdor. 2005. How C-type lectins detect pathogens. *Cell Microbiol.* **7:** 481–488.
16. van Vliet, S.J., J.J. Garcia-Vallejo & Y. van Kooyk. 2008. Dendritic cells and C-type lectin receptors: coupling innate to adaptive immune responses. *Immunol. Cell Biol.* **86:** 580–587.
17. Redelinghuys, P. & G.D. Brown. 2011. Inhibitory C-type lectin receptors in myeloid cells. *Immunol, Lett.* **136:** 1–12.
18. Akira, S. & K. Takeda. 2004. Toll-like receptor signalling. *Nat. Rev. Immunol.* **4:** 499–511.
19. Kato, H. *et al.* 2006. Differential roles of MDA5 and RIG-I helicases in the recognition of RNA viruses. *Nature* **441:** 101–105.
20. Pedra, J.H., S.L. Cassel & F.S. Sutterwala. 2009. Sensing pathogens and danger signals by the inflammasome. *Curr. Opin. Immunol.* **21:** 10–16.
21. Skoberne, M., A.S. Beignon & N. Bhardwaj. 2004. Danger signals: a time and space continuum. *Trends Mol. Med.* **10:** 251–257.
22. Jego, G. *et al.* 2005. Dendritic cells control B cell growth and differentiation. *Curr. Dir. Autoimmun.* **8:** 124–139.
23. Munz, C. *et al.* 2005. Mature myeloid dendritic cell subsets have distinct roles for activation and viability of circulating human natural killer cells. *Blood* **105:** 266–273.
24. Fujii, S. *et al.* 2002. Prolonged IFN-gamma-producing NKT response induced with alpha-galactosylceramide-loaded DCs. *Nat. Immunol.* **3:** 867–874.
25. Skoberne, M. *et al.* 2005. Apoptotic cells at the crossroads of tolerance and immunity. *Curr. Top. Microbiol. Immunol.* **289:** 259–292.
26. Cools, N. *et al.* 2007. Balancing between immunity and tolerance: an interplay between dendritic cells, regulatory T cells, and effector T cells. *J. Leukoc. Biol.* **82:** 1365–1374.
27. Mellor, A.L. & D.H. Munn. 2004. IDO expression by dendritic cells: tolerance and tryptophan catabolism. *Nat. Rev. Immunol.* **4:** 762–774.
28. Munn, D.H. & A.L. Mellor. 2004. IDO and tolerance to tumors. *Trends Mol. Med.* **10:** 15–18.
29. Levings, M.K. *et al.* 2005. Differentiation of Tr1 cells by immature dendritic cells requires IL-10 but not CD25$^+$CD4$^+$ Tr cells. *Blood* **105:** 1162–1169.
30. Jonuleit, H. *et al.* 2000. Induction of interleukin 10-producing, nonproliferating CD4(+) T cells with regulatory properties by repetitive stimulation with allogeneic immature human dendritic cells. *J. Exp. Med.* **192:** 1213–1222.
31. Woo, E.Y. *et al.* 2001. Regulatory CD4(+)CD25(+) T cells in tumors from patients with early-stage non-small cell

lung cancer and late-stage ovarian cancer. *Cancer Res.* **61:** 4766–4772.

32. Liyanage, U.K. *et al.* 2002. Prevalence of regulatory T cells is increased in peripheral blood and tumor microenvironment of patients with pancreas or breast adenocarcinoma. *J. Immunol.* **169:** 2756–2761.

33. Tang, Q. & J.A. Bluestone. 2008. The Foxp3+ regulatory T cell: a jack of all trades, master of regulation. *Nat. Immunol.* **9:** 239–244.

34. Skoberne, M. *et al.* 2006. The apoptotic-cell receptor CR3, but not alphavbeta5, is a regulator of human dendritic-cell immunostimulatory function. *Blood* **108:** 947–955.

35. Frleta, D. *et al.* 2012. HIV-1 infection-induced apoptotic microparticles inhibit human DCs via CD44. *J. Clin. Invest.* **122:** 4685–4697.

36. Agace, W.W. & E.K. Persson. 2012. How vitamin A metabolizing dendritic cells are generated in the gut mucosa. *Trends Immunol.* **33:** 42–48.

37. Satzger, I. *et al.* 2006. Spontaneous regression of melanoma with distant metastases—report of a patient with brain metastases. *Eur. J. Dermatol.* **16:** 454–455.

38. Wang, R.F. & S.A. Rosenberg. 1999. Human tumor antigens for cancer vaccine development. *Immunol. Rev.* **170:** 85–100.

39. Kim, R., M. Emi & K. Tanabe. 2007. Cancer immunoediting from immune surveillance to immune escape. *Immunology* **121:** 1–14.

40. Fridman, W.H. *et al.* 2012. The immune contexture in human tumours: impact on clinical outcome. Nature reviews. *Cancer* **12:** 298–306.

41. Sikora, A.G., Y. Hailemichael & W.W. Overwijk. 2012. Conference scene: immune effector mechanisms in tumor immunity. *Immunotherapy* **4:** 141–143.

42. Gandhi, R.T. *et al.* 2009. A randomized therapeutic vaccine trial of canarypox-HIV-pulsed dendritic cells vs. canarypox-HIV alone in HIV-1-infected patients on antiretroviral therapy. *Vaccine* **27:** 6088–6094.

43. Palucka, A.K. *et al.* 2006. Dendritic cells loaded with killed allogeneic melanoma cells can induce objective clinical responses and MART-1 specific CD8+ T-cell immunity. *J. Immunother.* **29:** 545–557.

44. Redman, B.G. *et al.* 2008. Phase Ib trial assessing autologous, tumor-pulsed dendritic cells as a vaccine administered with or without IL-2 in patients with metastatic melanoma. *J. Immunother.* **31:** 591–598.

45. O'Neill, D.W. & N. Bhardwaj. 2005. Differentiation of peripheral blood monocytes into dendritic cells. *Curr. Protoc. Immunol.* Chapter 22: Unit 22F 24.

46. O'Neill, D. & N. Bhardwaj. 2005. Generation of autologous peptide- and protein-pulsed dendritic cells for patient-specific immunotherapy. *Methods Mol. Med.* **109:** 97–112.

47. Bancereau, J. *et al.* 2001. Immune and clinical responses in patients with metastatic melanoma to CD34(+) progenitor-derived dendritic cell vaccine. *Cancer Res.* **61:** 6451–6458.

48. Klechevsky, E. *et al.* 2009. Understanding human myeloid dendritic cell subsets for the rational design of novel vaccines. *Hum. Immunol.* **70:** 281–288.

49. Romano, E. *et al.* 2011. Peptide-loaded Langerhans cells, despite increased IL15 secretion and T-cell activation in vitro, elicit antitumor T-cell responses comparable to peptide-loaded monocyte-derived dendritic cells in vivo. *Clin. Cancer Res.* **17:** 1984–1997.

50. Marroquin, C.E. *et al.* 2002. Mobilization of dendritic cell precursors in patients with cancer by flt3 ligand allows the generation of higher yields of cultured dendritic cells. *J. Immunother.* **25:** 278–288.

51. Pulendran, B. *et al.* 2000. Flt3-ligand and granulocyte colony-stimulating factor mobilize distinct human dendritic cell subsets in vivo. *J. Immunol.* **165:** 566–572.

52. Guimond, M. *et al.* 2010. In vivo role of Flt3 ligand and dendritic cells in NK cell homeostasis. *J. Immunol.* **184:** 2769–2775.

53. Kantoff, P.W. *et al.* 2010. Sipuleucel-T immunotherapy for castration-resistant prostate cancer. *N. Engl. J. Med.* **363:** 411–422.

54. Small, E.J. *et al.* 2006. Placebo-controlled phase III trial of immunologic therapy with sipuleucel-T (APC8015) in patients with metastatic, asymptomatic hormone refractory prostate cancer. *J. Clin. Oncol.* **24:** 3089–3094.

55. De Vries, I. J. *et al.* 2003. Effective migration of antigen-pulsed dendritic cells to lymph nodes in melanoma patients is determined by their maturation state. *Cancer Res.* **63:** 12–17.

56. Dhodapkar, M.V. *et al.* 2001. Antigen-specific inhibition of effector T cell function in humans after injection of immature dendritic cells. *J. Exp. Med.* **193:** 233–238.

57. Dhodapkar, M.V. & R.M. Steinman. 2002. Antigen-bearing immature dendritic cells induce peptide-specific CD8(+) regulatory T cells in vivo in humans. *Blood* **100:** 174–177.

58. de Vries, I.J. *et al.* 2003. Maturation of dendritic cells is a prerequisite for inducing immune responses in advanced melanoma patients. *Clin. Cancer Res.* **9:** 5091–5100.

59. Lee, A.W. *et al.* 2002. A clinical grade cocktail of cytokines and PGE2 results in uniform maturation of human monocyte-derived dendritic cells: implications for immunotherapy. *Vaccine* **20** (Suppl. 4): A8–A22.

60. Jongmans, W. *et al.* 2005. Th1-polarizing capacity of clinical-grade dendritic cells is triggered by Ribomunyl but is compromised by PGE2: the importance of maturation cocktails. *J. Immunother.* **28:** 480–487.

61. Krause, P. *et al.* 2007. Prostaglandin E2 is a key factor for monocyte-derived dendritic cell maturation: enhanced T cell stimulatory capacity despite IDO. *J. Leukoc. Biol.* **82:** 1106–1114.

62. Morelli, A.E. & A.W. Thomson. 2003. Dendritic cells under the spell of prostaglandins. *Trends Immunol.* **24:** 108–111.

63. Baratelli, F.E. *et al.* 2004. Prostaglandin E2-dependent enhancement of tissue inhibitors of metalloproteinases-1 production limits dendritic cell migration through extracellular matrix. *J. Immunol.* **173:** 5458–5466.

64. Scandella, E. *et al.* 2002. Prostaglandin E2 is a key factor for CCR7 surface expression and migration of monocyte-derived dendritic cells. *Blood* **100:** 1354–1361.

65. Krause, P. *et al.* 2009. Prostaglandin E(2) enhances T-cell proliferation by inducing the costimulatory molecules OX40L, CD70, and 4–1BBL on dendritic cells. *Blood* **113:** 2451–2460.

66. Kwissa, M. *et al.* 2012. Distinct TLR adjuvants differentially stimulate systemic and local innate immune responses in nonhuman primates. *Blood* 119: 2044–2055.

67. Schnare, M. *et al.* 2001. Toll-like receptors control activation of adaptive immune responses. *Nat. Immunol.* 2: 947–950.

68. Napolitani, G. *et al.* 2005. Selected Toll-like receptor agonist combinations synergistically trigger a T helper type 1-polarizing program in dendritic cells. *Nat. Immunol.* 6: 769–776.

69. Boullart, A.C. *et al.* 2008. Maturation of monocyte-derived dendritic cells with Toll-like receptor 3 and 7/8 ligands combined with prostaglandin E2 results in high interleukin-12 production and cell migration. *Cancer Immunol. Immunother.* 57: 1589–1597.

70. Mailliard, R.B. *et al.* 2004. alpha-type-1 polarized dendritic cells: a novel immunization tool with optimized CTL-inducing activity. *Cancer Res.* 64: 5934–5937.

71. Lee, J.J. *et al.* 2008. Type 1-polarized dendritic cells loaded with autologous tumor are a potent immunogen against chronic lymphocytic leukemia. *J. Leukoc. Biol.* 84: 319–325.

72. Okada, H. *et al.* 2011. Induction of CD8[+] T-cell responses against novel glioma-associated antigen peptides and clinical activity by vaccinations with {alpha}-type 1 polarized dendritic cells and polyinosinic-polycytidylic acid stabilized by lysine and carboxymethylcellulose in patients with recurrent malignant glioma. *J. Clin. Oncol.* 29: 330–336.

73. MartIn-Fontecha, A. *et al.* 2003. Regulation of dendritic cell migration to the draining lymph node: impact on T lymphocyte traffic and priming. *J. Exp. Med.* 198: 615–621.

74. Adams, S. *et al.* 2008. Immunization of malignant melanoma patients with full-length NY-ESO-1 protein using TLR7 agonist imiquimod as vaccine adjuvant. *J. Immunol.* 181: 776–784.

75. Nair, S. *et al.* 2003. Injection of immature dendritic cells into adjuvant-treated skin obviates the need for ex vivo maturation. *J. Immunol.* 171: 6275–6282.

76. Melief, C.J. & S.H. van der Burg. 2008. Immunotherapy of established (pre)malignant disease by synthetic long peptide vaccines. *Nat. Rev. Cancer* 8: 351–360.

77. Bijker, M.S. *et al.* 2008. Superior induction of anti-tumor CTL immunity by extended peptide vaccines involves prolonged, DC-focused antigen presentation. *Eur. J. Immunol.* 38: 1033–1042.

78. Kenter, G.G. *et al.* 2008. Phase I immunotherapeutic trial with long peptides spanning the E6 and E7 sequences of high-risk human papillomavirus 16 in end-stage cervical cancer patients shows low toxicity and robust immunogenicity. *Clin. Cancer Res.* 14: 169–177.

79. Welters, M.J. *et al.* 2008. Induction of tumor-specific CD4[+] and CD8[+] T-cell immunity in cervical cancer patients by a human papillomavirus type 16 E6 and E7 long peptides vaccine. *Clin. Cancer Res.* 14: 178–187.

80. Kenter, G.G. *et al.* 2009. Vaccination against HPV-16 oncoproteins for vulvar intraepithelial neoplasia. *N. Engl. J. Med.* 361: 1838–1847.

81. de Vos van Steenwijk, P.J. *et al.* 2012. A placebo-controlled randomized HPV16 synthetic long-peptide vaccination study in women with high-grade cervical squamous intraepithelial lesions. *Cancer Immunol. Immunother.* 61: 1485–1492.

82. Leffers, N. *et al.* 2009. Immunization with a P53 synthetic long peptide vaccine induces P53-specific immune responses in ovarian cancer patients, a phase II trial. *Int. J. Cancer* 125: 2104–2113.

83. Sabbatini, P. *et al.* 2012. Phase I trial of overlapping long peptides from a tumor self-antigen and poly-ICLC shows rapid induction of integrated immune response in ovarian cancer patients. *Clin. Cancer Res.* 18: 6497–6508.

84. Zeestraten, E.C. *et al.* 2013. Addition of interferon-alpha to the p53-SLP(R) vaccine results in increased production of interferon-gamma in vaccinated colorectal cancer patients: a phase I/II clinical trial. *Int. J. Cancer* 132: 1581–1591.

85. Speetjens, F.M. *et al.* 2009. Induction of p53-specific immunity by a p53 synthetic long peptide vaccine in patients treated for metastatic colorectal cancer. *Clin. Cancer Res.* 15: 1086–1095.

86. Rosario, M. *et al.* 2012. Prime-boost regimens with adjuvanted synthetic long peptides elicit T cells and antibodies to conserved regions of HIV-1 in macaques. *Aids* 26: 275–284.

87. Barrou, B. *et al.* 2004. Vaccination of prostatectomized prostate cancer patients in biochemical relapse, with autologous dendritic cells pulsed with recombinant human PSA. *Cancer Immunol. Immunother.* 53: 453–460.

88. Salcedo, M. *et al.* 2006. Vaccination of melanoma patients using dendritic cells loaded with an allogeneic tumor cell lysate. *Cancer Immunol. Immunother.* 55: 819–829.

89. Mahdian, R. *et al.* 2006. Dendritic cells, pulsed with lysate of allogeneic tumor cells, are capable of stimulating MHC-restricted antigen-specific antitumor T cells. *Med. Oncol.* 23: 273–282.

90. Schnurr, M. *et al.* 2001. Tumor cell lysate-pulsed human dendritic cells induce a T-cell response against pancreatic carcinoma cells: an in vitro model for the assessment of tumor vaccines. *Cancer Res.* 61: 6445–6450.

91. Thumann, P. *et al.* 2003. Antigen loading of dendritic cells with whole tumor cell preparations. *J. Immunol. Methods* 277: 1–16.

92. Knutson, K.L. 2002. Technology evaluation: DCVax, Northwest Biotherapeutics. *Curr. Opin. Mol. Ther.* 4: 403–407.

93. Kandalaft, L.E. *et al.* 2013. Autologous lysate-pulsed dendritic cell vaccination followed by adoptive transfer of vaccine-primed ex vivo co-stimulated T cells in recurrent ovarian cancer. *Oncoimmunology* 2: e22664.

94. Schnurr, M. *et al.* 2005. Tumor antigen processing and presentation depend critically on dendritic cell type and the mode of antigen delivery. *Blood* 105: 2465–2472.

95. Jenne, L., G. Schuler & A. Steinkasserer. 2001. Viral vectors for dendritic cell-based immunotherapy. *Trends Immunol.* 22: 102–107.

96. Brockstedt, D.G. & T.W. Dubensky. 2008. Promises and challenges for the development of Listeria monocytogenes-based immunotherapies. *Expert Rev. Vaccines* 7: 1069–1084.

97. Bellone, S. *et al.* 2009. Human papillomavirus type 16 (HPV-16) virus-like particle L1-specific CD8+ cytotoxic T lymphocytes (CTLs) are equally effective as E7-specific

CD8+ CTLs in killing autologous HPV-16-positive tumor cells in cervical cancer patients: implications for L1 dendritic cell-based therapeutic vaccines. *J. Virol.* **83:** 6779–6789.

98. Carrasco, J. *et al.* 2008. Vaccination of a melanoma patient with mature dendritic cells pulsed with MAGE-3 peptides triggers the activity of nonvaccine anti-tumor cells. *J. Immunol.* **180:** 3585–3593.

99. Butterfield, L.H. *et al.* 2008. Adenovirus MART-1-engineered autologous dendritic cell vaccine for metastatic melanoma. *J. Immunother.* **31:** 294–309.

100. Veron, P. *et al.* 2007. Major subsets of human dendritic cells are efficiently transduced by self-complementary adeno-associated virus vectors 1 and 2. *J. Virol.* **81:** 5385–5394.

101. Skoberne, M. *et al.* 2008. KBMA Listeria monocytogenes is an effective vector for DC-mediated induction of antitumor immunity. *J. Clin. Invest.* **118:** 3990–4001.

102. Breckpot, K., J.L. Aerts & K. Thielemans. 2007. Lentiviral vectors for cancer immunotherapy: transforming infectious particles into therapeutics. *Gene Ther.* **14:** 847–862.

103. He, Y., D. Munn & L.D. Falo Jr. 2007. Recombinant lentivector as a genetic immunization vehicle for antitumor immunity. *Expert Rev. Vaccines.* **6:** 913–924.

104. Schroers, R. *et al.* 2000. Transduction of human PBMC-derived dendritic cells and macrophages by an HIV-1-based lentiviral vector system. *Mol. Ther.* **1:** 171–179.

105. Dyall, J. *et al.* 2001. Lentivirus-transduced human monocyte-derived dendritic cells efficiently stimulate antigen-specific cytotoxic T lymphocytes. *Blood* **97:** 114–121.

106. Lizee, G., M.I. Gonzales & S.L. Topalian. 2004. Lentivirus vector-mediated expression of tumor-associated epitopes by human antigen presenting cells. *Hum. Gene Ther.* **15:** 393–404.

107. Bobadilla, S., N. Sunseri & N.R. Landau. 2012. Efficient transduction of myeloid cells by an HIV-1-derived lentiviral vector that packages the Vpx accessory protein. *Gene Ther.*

108. Breckpot, K. *et al.* 2004. Identification of new antigenic peptide presented by HLA-Cw7 and encoded by several MAGE genes using dendritic cells transduced with lentiviruses. *J. Immunol.* **172:** 2232–2237.

109. He, Y. *et al.* 2005. Immunization with lentiviral vector-transduced dendritic cells induces strong and long-lasting T cell responses and therapeutic immunity. *J. Immunol.* **174:** 3808–3817.

110. Dullaers, M. *et al.* 2006. Induction of effective therapeutic antitumor immunity by direct in vivo administration of lentiviral vectors. *Gene Ther.* **13:** 630–640.

111. Yang, L. *et al.* 2008. Engineered lentivector targeting of dendritic cells for in vivo immunization. *Nat. Biotechnol.* **26:** 326–334.

112. Nair, S.K. *et al.* 2002. Induction of tumor-specific cytotoxic T lymphocytes in cancer patients by autologous tumor RNA-transfected dendritic cells. *Ann. Surg.* **235:** 540–549.

113. Muller, M.R. *et al.* 2004. Induction of chronic lymphocytic leukemia (CLL)-specific CD4- and CD8-mediated T-cell responses using RNA-transfected dendritic cells. *Blood* **103:** 1763–1769.

114. Nencioni, A. *et al.* 2003. Dendritic cells transfected with tumor RNA for the induction of antitumor CTL in colorectal cancer. *Cancer Gene Ther.* **10:** 209–214.

115. Milazzo, C. *et al.* 2003. Induction of myeloma-specific cytotoxic T cells using dendritic cells transfected with tumor-derived RNA. *Blood* **101:** 977–982.

116. Gilboa, E. & J. Vieweg. 2004. Cancer immunotherapy with mRNA-transfected dendritic cells. *Immunol. Rev.* **199:** 251–263.

117. Heiser, A. *et al.* 2001. Human dendritic cells transfected with renal tumor RNA stimulate polyclonal T-cell responses against antigens expressed by primary and metastatic tumors. *Cancer Res.* **61:** 3388–3393.

118. Strobel, I. *et al.* 2000. Human dendritic cells transfected with either RNA or DNA encoding influenza matrix protein M1 differ in their ability to stimulate cytotoxic T lymphocytes. *Gene Ther.* **7:** 2028–2035.

119. Koido, S. *et al.* 2000. Induction of antitumor immunity by vaccination of dendritic cells transfected with MUC1 RNA. *J. Immunol.* **165:** 5713–5719.

120. Heiser, A. *et al.* 2002. Autologous dendritic cells transfected with prostate-specific antigen RNA stimulate CTL responses against metastatic prostate tumors. *J. Clin. Invest.* **109:** 409–417.

121. Routy, J.P. *et al.* 2010. Immunologic activity and safety of autologous HIV RNA-electroporated dendritic cells in HIV-1 infected patients receiving antiretroviral therapy. *Clin. Immunol.* **134:** 140–147.

122. Shortman, K., M.H. Lahoud & I. Caminschi. 2009. Improving vaccines by targeting antigens to dendritic cells. *Exp. Mol. Med.* **41:** 61–66.

123. Tacken, P.J., R. Torensma & C.G. Figdor. 2006. Targeting antigens to dendritic cells in vivo. *Immunobiology* **211:** 599–608.

124. Jinushi, M., F.S. Hodi & G. Dranoff. 2008. Enhancing the clinical activity of granulocyte-macrophage colony-stimulating factor-secreting tumor cell vaccines. *Immunol. Rev.* **222:** 287–298.

125. Jinushi, M. & H. Tahara. 2009. Cytokine gene-mediated immunotherapy: current status and future perspectives. *Cancer Sci.* **100:** 1389–1396.

126. Filipazzi, P. *et al.* 2007. Identification of a new subset of myeloid suppressor cells in peripheral blood of melanoma patients with modulation by a granulocyte-macrophage colony-stimulation factor-based antitumor vaccine. *J. Clin. Oncol.* **25:** 2546–2553.

127. Sica, A. & V. Bronte. 2007. Altered macrophage differentiation and immune dysfunction in tumor development. *J. Clin. Invest.* **117:** 1155–1166.

128. Lutz, E. *et al.* 2011. A lethally irradiated allogeneic granulocyte-macrophage colony stimulating factor-secreting tumor vaccine for pancreatic adenocarcinoma. A phase II trial of safety, efficacy, and immune activation. *Ann. Surg.* **253:** 328–335.

129. Bayne, L.J. *et al.* 2012. Tumor-derived granulocyte-macrophage colony-stimulating factor regulates myeloid inflammation and T cell immunity in pancreatic cancer. *Cancer Cell.* **21:** 822–835.

130. van Kooyk, Y. 2008. C-type lectins on dendritic cells: key modulators for the induction of immune responses. *Biochem. Soc. Trans.* **36:** 1478–1481.

131. Caminschi, I. *et al.* 2008. The dendritic cell subtype-restricted C-type lectin Clec9A is a target for vaccine enhancement. *Blood* **112:** 3264–3273.

132. Carter, R.W. *et al.* 2006. Preferential induction of CD4$^+$ T cell responses through in vivo targeting of antigen to dendritic cell-associated C-type lectin-1. *J. Immunol.* **177:** 2276–2284.

133. Carter, R.W. *et al.* 2006. Induction of CD8$^+$ T cell responses through targeting of antigen to Dectin-2. *Cell Immunol.* **239:** 87–91.

134. Boscardin, S.B. *et al.* 2006. Antigen targeting to dendritic cells elicits long-lived T cell help for antibody responses. *J. Exp. Med.* **203:** 599–606.

135. Wang, B. *et al.* 2012. Targeting of the non-mutated tumor antigen HER2/neu to mature dendritic cells induces an integrated immune response that protects against breast cancer in mice. *Breast Cancer Res.* **14:** R39.

136. Cheong, C. *et al.* 2010. Improved cellular and humoral immune responses in vivo following targeting of HIV Gag to dendritic cells within human anti-human DEC205 monoclonal antibody. *Blood* **116:** 3828–3838.

137. Idoyaga, J. *et al.* 2011. Comparable T helper 1 (Th1) and CD8 T-cell immunity by targeting HIV gag p24 to CD8 dendritic cells within antibodies to Langerin, DEC205, and Clec9A. *Proc. Natl. Acad. Sci. US A* **108:** 2384–2389.

138. Tacken, P.J. *et al.* 2005. Effective induction of naive and recall T-cell responses by targeting antigen to human dendritic cells via a humanized anti-DC-SIGN antibody. *Blood* **106:** 1278–1285.

139. Ramakrishna, V. *et al.* 2004. Mannose receptor targeting of tumor antigen pmel17 to human dendritic cells directs anti-melanoma T cell responses via multiple HLA molecules. *J. Immunol.* **172:** 2845–2852.

140. Trumpfheller, C. *et al.* 2012. Dendritic cell-targeted protein vaccines: a novel approach to induce T-cell immunity. *J. Intern. Med.* **271:** 183–192.

141. Verdijk, P. *et al.* 2009. Limited amounts of dendritic cells migrate into the T-cell area of lymph nodes but have high immune activating potential in melanoma patients. *Clin. Cancer Res.* **15:** 2531–2540.

142. Fujiwara, S. *et al.* 2012. Clinical trial of the intratumoral administration of labeled DC combined with systemic chemotherapy for esophageal cancer. *J. Immunother.* **35:** 513–521.

143. Lesterhuis, W.J. *et al.* 2011. Route of administration modulates the induction of dendritic cell vaccine-induced antigen-specific T cells in advanced melanoma patients. *Clin. Cancer Res.* **17:** 5725–5735.

144. Aarntzen, E.H. *et al.* 2013. Targeting of 111In-labeled dendritic cell human vaccines improved by reducing number of cells. *Clin. Cancer Res.* **19:** 1525–1533

145. Yewdall, A.W. *et al.* 2010. CD8$^+$ T cell priming by dendritic cell vaccines requires antigen transfer to endogenous antigen presenting cells. *PLoS One* **5:** e11144.

146. Schadendorf, D. *et al.* 2006. Dacarbazine (DTIC) versus vaccination with autologous peptide-pulsed dendritic cells (DC) in first-line treatment of patients with metastatic melanoma: a randomized phase III trial of the DC study group of the DeCOG. *Ann. Oncol.* **17:** 563–570.

147. Higano, C.S. *et al.* 2009. Integrated data from 2 randomized, double-blind, placebo-controlled, phase 3 trials of active cellular immunotherapy with sipuleucel-T in advanced prostate cancer. *Cancer* **115:** 3670–3679.

148. Bennaceur, K. *et al.* 2008. Dendritic cells dysfunction in tumour environment. *Cancer Lett.* **272:** 186–196.

149. Aptsiauri, N. *et al.* 2007. Role of altered expression of HLA class I molecules in cancer progression. *Adv. Exp. Med. Biol.* **601:** 123–131.

150. Bronte, V. & S. Mocellin. 2009. Suppressive influences in the immune response to cancer. *J. Immunother.* **32:** 1–11.

151. Chang, C.C. *et al.* 2006. Defective human leukocyte antigen class I-associated antigen presentation caused by a novel beta2-microglobulin loss-of-function in melanoma cells. *J. Biol. Chem.* **281:** 18763–18773.

152. Peggs, K.S. *et al.* 2009. Blockade of CTLA-4 on both effector and regulatory T cell compartments contributes to the antitumor activity of anti-CTLA-4 antibodies. *J. Exp. Med.* **206:** 1717–1725.

153. Pardoll, D.M. 2012. The blockade of immune checkpoints in cancer immunotherapy. Nature reviews. *Cancer* **12:** 252–264.

154. Iwai, Y. *et al.* 2002. Involvement of PD-L1 on tumor cells in the escape from host immune system and tumor immunotherapy by PD-L1 blockade. *Proc. Natl. Acad. Sci. USA* **99:** 12293–12297.

155. Strome, S.E. *et al.* 2003. B7-H1 blockade augments adoptive T-cell immunotherapy for squamous cell carcinoma. *Cancer Res.* **63:** 6501–6505.

156. Blank, C. *et al.* 2006. Blockade of PD-L1 (B7-H1) augments human tumor-specific T cell responses in vitro. *Int. J. Cancer* **119:** 317–327.

157. Berger, R. *et al.* 2008. Phase I safety and pharmacokinetic study of CT-011, a humanized antibody interacting with PD-1, in patients with advanced hematologic malignancies. *Clin. Cancer Res.* **14:** 3044–3051.

158. Brahmer, J.R. *et al.* 2010. Phase I study of single-agent anti-programmed death-1 (MDX-1106) in refractory solid tumors: safety, clinical activity, pharmacodynamics, and immunologic correlates. *J. Clin. Oncol.* **28:** 3167–3175.

159. Topalian, S.L. *et al.* 2012. Safety, activity, and immune correlates of anti-PD-1 antibody in cancer. *N. Engl. J. Med.* **366:** 2443–2454.

160. Brahmer, J.R. *et al.* 2012. Safety and activity of anti-PD-L1 antibody in patients with advanced cancer. *N. Engl. J. Med.* **366:** 2455–2465.

161. Yuan, J. *et al.* 2008. CTLA-4 blockade enhances polyfunctional NY-ESO-1 specific T cell responses in metastatic melanoma patients with clinical benefit. *Proc. Natl. Acad. Sci. USA* **105:** 20410–20415.

162. Hodi, F.S. *et al.* 2010. Improved survival with ipilimumab in patients with metastatic melanoma. *N. Engl. J. Med.* **363:** 711–723.

163. O'Day, S.J., O. Hamid & W.J. Urba. 2007. Targeting cytotoxic T-lymphocyte antigen-4 (CTLA-4): a novel strategy

for the treatment of melanoma and other malignancies. *Cancer* **110:** 2614–2627.

164. Wang, C. *et al.* 2009. Immune regulation by 4–1BB and 4–1BBL: complexities and challenges. *Immunol. Rev.* **229:** 192–215.

165. May, K.F., Jr. *et al.* 2002. Anti-4–1BB monoclonal antibody enhances rejection of large tumor burden by promoting survival but not clonal expansion of tumor-specific CD8$^+$ T cells. *Cancer Res.* **62:** 3459–3465.

166. Murillo, O. *et al.* 2009. In vivo depletion of DC impairs the anti-tumor effect of agonistic anti-CD137 mAb. *Eur. J. Immunol.* **39:** 2424–2436.

167. Kocak, E. *et al.* 2006. Combination therapy with anti-CTL antigen-4 and anti-4–1BB antibodies enhances cancer immunity and reduces autoimmunity. *Cancer Res.* **66:** 7276–7284.

168. Simeone, E. & P.A. Ascierto. 2012. Immunomodulating antibodies in the treatment of metastatic melanoma: the experience with anti-CTLA-4, anti-CD137, and anti-PD1. *J. Immunotoxicol.* **9:** 241–247.

169. Elgueta, R. *et al.* 2009. Molecular mechanism and function of CD40/CD40L engagement in the immune system. *Immunol. Rev.* **229:** 152–172.

170. Vonderheide, R.H. & M.J. Glennie. 2013. Agonistic CD40 antibodies and cancer therapy. *Clin. Cancer Res.* **19:** 1035–1043.

171. Beatty, G.L. *et al.* 2011. CD40 agonists alter tumor stroma and show efficacy against pancreatic carcinoma in mice and humans. *Science* **331:** 1612–1616.

172. Kutzler, M.A. *et al.* 2005. Coimmunization with an optimized IL-15 plasmid results in enhanced function and longevity of CD8 T cells that are partially independent of CD4 T cell help. *J. Immunol.* **175:** 112–123.

173. Klebanoff, C.A. *et al.* 2004. IL-15 enhances the in vivo antitumor activity of tumor-reactive CD8$^+$ T cells. *Proc. Natl. Acad. Sci. USA* **101:** 1969–1974.

174. Teague, R.M. *et al.* 2006. Interleukin-15 rescues tolerant CD8$^+$ T cells for use in adoptive immunotherapy of established tumors. *Nat. Med.* **12:** 335–341.

175. Steel, J.C., T.A. Waldmann & J.C. Morris. 2012. Interleukin-15 biology and its therapeutic implications in cancer. *Trends Pharmacol. Sci.* **33:** 35–41.

176. Pouw, N. *et al.* 2010. Combination of IL-21 and IL-15 enhances tumour-specific cytotoxicity and cytokine production of TCR-transduced primary T cells. *Cancer Immunol. Immunother.* **59:** 921–931.

177. Jakobisiak, M., J. Golab & W. Lasek. 2011. Interleukin 15 as a promising candidate for tumor immunotherapy. *Cytok. Growth Factor Rev.* **22:** 99–108.

178. Schluns, K.S. *et al.* 2000. Interleukin-7 mediates the homeostasis of naive and memory CD8 T cells in vivo. *Nat. Immunol.* **1:** 426–432.

179. Rosenberg, S.A. *et al.* 2006. IL-7 administration to humans leads to expansion of CD8$^+$ and CD4$^+$ cells but a relative decrease of CD4$^+$ T regulatory cells. *J. Immunother.* **29:** 313–319.

180. Minkis, K. *et al.* 2008. Type 2 Bias of T cells expanded from the blood of melanoma patients switched to type 1 by IL-12p70 mRNA-transfected dendritic cells. *Cancer Res.* **68:** 9441–9450.

181. Trinchieri, G. 2003. Interleukin-12 and the regulation of innate resistance and adaptive immunity. *Nat. Rev. Immunol.* **3:** 133–146.

182. Czerniecki, B.J. *et al.* 2007. Targeting HER-2/neu in early breast cancer development using dendritic cells with staged interleukin-12 burst secretion. *Cancer Res.* **67:** 1842–1852.

183. Rudman, S.M. *et al.* 2011. A phase 1 study of AS1409, a novel antibody-cytokine fusion protein, in patients with malignant melanoma or renal cell carcinoma. *Clin. Cancer Res.* **17:** 1998–2005.

184. Vicari, A.P. *et al.* 2002. Reversal of tumor-induced dendritic cell paralysis by CpG immunostimulatory oligonucleotide and anti-interleukin 10 receptor antibody. *J. Exp. Med.* **196:** 541–549.

185. Fujita, T. *et al.* 2009. Inhibition of transforming growth factor-beta-mediated immunosuppression in tumor-draining lymph nodes augments antitumor responses by various immunologic cell types. *Cancer Res.* **69:** 5142–5150.

186. Lopez, M.N. *et al.* 2009. Prolonged survival of dendritic cell-vaccinated melanoma patients correlates with tumor-specific delayed type IV hypersensitivity response and reduction of tumor growth factor beta-expressing T cells. *J. Clin. Oncol.* **27:** 945–952.

187. Speiser, D.E. *et al.* 2005. Rapid and strong human CD8$^+$ T cell responses to vaccination with peptide, IFA, and CpG oligodeoxynucleotide 7909. *J. Clin. Invest.* **115:** 739–746.

188. Longhi, M.P. *et al.* 2009. Dendritic cells require a systemic type I interferon response to mature and induce CD4$^+$ Th1 immunity with poly IC as adjuvant. *J. Exp. Med.* **206:** 1589–1602.

189. Warger, T. *et al.* 2006. Synergistic activation of dendritic cells by combined Toll-like receptor ligation induces superior CTL responses in vivo. *Blood* **108:** 544–550.

190. Vandepapeliere, P. *et al.* 2008. Vaccine adjuvant systems containing monophosphoryl lipid A and QS21 induce strong and persistent humoral and T cell responses against hepatitis B surface antigen in healthy adult volunteers. *Vaccine* **26:** 1375–1386.

191. Baumgaertner, P. *et al.* 2006. Ex vivo detectable human CD8 T-cell responses to cancer-testis antigens. *Cancer Res.* **66:** 1912–1916.

192. Diefenbach, C.S. *et al.* 2008. Safety and immunogenicity study of NY-ESO-1b peptide and montanide ISA-51 vaccination of patients with epithelial ovarian cancer in high-risk first remission. *Clin. Cancer Res.* **14:** 2740–2748.

193. Fourcade, J. *et al.* 2008. Immunization with analog peptide in combination with CpG and montanide expands tumor antigen-specific CD8+ T cells in melanoma patients. *J. Immunother.* **31:** 781–791.

194. Dhodapkar, M.V. 2009. Harnessing human CD1d restricted T cells for tumor immunity: progress and challenges. *Front. Biosci.* **14:** 796–807.

195. Chang, D.H. *et al.* 2005. Sustained expansion of NKT cells and antigen-specific T cells after injection of alpha-galactosyl-ceramide loaded mature dendritic cells in cancer patients. *J. Exp. Med.* **201:** 1503–1517.

196. Marshall, J.L. *et al.* 2005. Phase I study of sequential vaccinations with fowlpox-CEA(6D)-TRICOM alone and sequentially with vaccinia-CEA(6D)-TRICOM, with and without granulocyte-macrophage colony-stimulating factor, in patients with carcinoembryonic antigen-expressing carcinomas. *J. Clin. Oncol.* **23:** 720–731.

197. Marshall, J.L. *et al.* 2000. Phase I study in advanced cancer patients of a diversified prime-and-boost vaccination protocol using recombinant vaccinia virus and recombinant nonreplicating avipox virus to elicit anti-carcinoembryonic antigen immune responses. *J. Clin. Oncol.* **18:** 3964–3973.

198. Kaneno, R. *et al.* 2009. Chemomodulation of human dendritic cell function by antineoplastic agents in low noncytotoxic concentrations. *J. Transl. Med.* **7:** 58.

199. Shurin, G.V. *et al.* 2009. Chemotherapeutic agents in noncytotoxic concentrations increase antigen presentation by dendritic cells via an IL-12-dependent mechanism. *J. Immunol.* **183:** 137–144.

200. Aquino, A. *et al.* 2004. Drug-induced increase of carcinoembryonic antigen expression in cancer cells. *Pharmacol. Res.* **49:** 383–396.

201. Correale, P. *et al.* 2003. Treatment of colon and breast carcinoma cells with 5-fluorouracil enhances expression of carcinoembryonic antigen and susceptibility to HLA-A(*)02.01 restricted, CEA-peptide-specific cytotoxic T cells in vitro. *Int. J. Cancer* **104:** 437–445.

202. Kikuta, J. & M. Ishii. 2012. Recent advances in intravital imaging of dynamic biological systems. *J. Pharmacol. Sci.* **119:** 193–197.

203. Lu, W. *et al.* 2004. Therapeutic dendritic-cell vaccine for chronic HIV-1 infection. *Nat. Med.* **10:** 1359–1365.

204. Garcia, F. *et al.* 2013. A dendritic cell-based vaccine elicits T cell responses associated with control of HIV-1 replication. *Sci. Transl. Med.* **5:** 166ra162.

Ann. N.Y. Acad. Sci. ISSN 0077-8923

Molecular programming of steady-state dendritic cells: impact on autoimmunity and tumor immune surveillance

Dylan J. Johnson[1,2] and Pamela S. Ohashi[1,2,3]

[1]Campbell Family Institute for Breast Cancer Research, Princess Margaret Cancer Center, University Health Network. [2]Department of Immunology. [3]Department of Medical Biophysics, University of Toronto, Toronto, Ontario, Canada

Address for correspondence: Pamela Ohashi, Ph.D., Princess Margaret Hospital, 10th Floor Rm. 1030, 620 University Ave., Toronto, ON, Canada M5G 2C1. pohashi@uhnresearch.ca

Dendritic cells are master regulators of immunity. Immature dendritic cells are essential for maintaining self-tolerance, while mature dendritic cells initiate a variety of specialized immune responses. Dendritic cell quiescence is often viewed as a default state that requires exogenous stimuli to induce maturation. However, recent studies have identified dendritic cell quiescence factors that actively program dendritic cells to an immature state. In the absence of these factors, dendritic cells spontaneously become immunogenic and can induce autoimmune responses. Herein we discuss two such factors, NF-κB1 and A20, that preserve dendritic cell immaturity through their regulation of NF-κB signaling. Loss of either of these factors increases dendritic cell immunogenicity, suggesting that they may be important targets for enhancing dendritic cell–based cancer immunotherapies. Alternatively, defects in molecules critical for maintaining steady-state DCs may provide novel biomarkers that identify patients who have enhanced natural antitumor immunity or that correlate with better responses to various immunotherapies.

Keywords: dendritic cells; immunotherapy; NF-κB

Dendritic cells control T cell tolerance and immunity

Dendritic cells (DCs) are at the crux of the immune system, regulating the induction of both tolerance and immunity. They act as sentinels, detecting molecular patterns associated with infection and injury, and acquiring self and foreign antigen to present to lymphocytes. Through their role as professional antigen presenting cells (APCs), DCs control T cell activation, and thereby promote or restrict inflammation. DCs are a heterogeneous population of cells that can be broadly divided into two major categories: conventional DCs (cDCs), which are exceptionally potent APCs and are the focus of this review, and plasmacytoid DCs (pDCs), which are noted for their ability to produce large amounts of type I interferon.

DCs are essential for T cell tolerance, which is highlighted by the finding that mice lacking both cDCs and pDCs develop systemic autoimmunity.[1]

DCs play a role in promoting both central and peripheral tolerance. Thymic DCs have been shown to play a role in negative selection and the development of regulatory T (T_{reg}) cells, while peripheral DCs can promote tolerance to soluble or apoptotic cell-derived self-antigen through the induction of T cell anergy or deletion. Additionally, DCs can induce the differentiation of peripheral T cells into T_{reg} cells. Despite their importance in tolerance, DCs also have a critical and well-established role in the initiation of immune responses to infection and cancer.[2] They can efficiently prime both CD4$^+$ and CD8$^+$ T cells, polarize immune responses, and promote the maintenance of T cell memory.

These seemingly discordant DC functions are consequences of their tightly regulated maturation. Under homeostatic conditions, DCs are found primarily with an immature or tolerogenic phenotype; they have high endocyotic activity, facilitating antigen acquisition, and yet express low levels of major histocompatibility class II (MHCII)

doi: 10.1111/nyas.12114

and T cell costimulatory molecules such as CD80 and CD86, thereby limiting their immunogenicity. Consequently, interaction between a functionally immature DC and a T cell results in tolerance, through T cell clonal deletion, anergy, or T_{reg} cell generation. However, DC maturation can be induced by numerous stimuli, including activation of pathogen-associated molecular pattern (PAMP) receptors such as Toll-like receptors (TLRs), NOD-like receptors (NLRs), RIG-like receptors (RLRs), and C-type lectin receptors, which may be expressed by immature DCs.

DC stimulation upregulates surface expression of of MHCII, CD80, and CD86, as well as the production of cytokines such as IL-6, TNF-α, and IL-12. Mature DCs have an immunogenic phenotype and therefore can induce T cell activation. The conventional paradigm of DC maturation suggests that DC immaturity is a default steady state and that activation through exogenous signals (e.g., ligation of TLRs) is required to initiate DC maturation. However, recent evidence suggests that DC immaturity is an active program that requires tight regulation of NF-κB family members. Dysregulation of the NF-κB signaling axis can result in functional maturation of DCs in the absence of exogenous stimuli.

DC stimulation activates NF-κB signaling

The NF-κB family of transcription factors is central to the mammalian immune system, mediating effects downstream of many receptors for antigens, cytokines, and PAMPs.[3] There are five members of the NF-κB family: NF-κB1, which includes p50 and its precursor protein p105; NF-κB2, which includes p52 and its precursor protein p100; RelA (p65); RelB; and c-Rel. All seven NF-κB proteins contain a Rel homology domain (RHD) that mediates the homo- and heterodimerization of NF-κB proteins. NF-κB dimers regulate gene expression by binding κB sites within DNA, where they either block or initiate gene transcription. RelA, RelB, and c-Rel contain transactivation domains, and dimers containing these proteins can therefore drive transcription directly. By contrast, p50 and p52 do not contain transactivation domains; dimers containing only p50 and/or p52 are therefore unable to directly activate transcription. NF-κB signaling is often divided into two discrete pathways: the canonical pathway downstream of TLRs and cytokine receptors that

activates RelA, c-Rel, and p50; and the noncanonical pathway downstream of LTβR and CD40, which activates RelB and p52. However, recent evidence suggests that this dichotomy may not hold true in DCs and that RelB may participate in signaling from TLRs.[4]

NF-κB activity is tightly regulated. In unstimulated cells, NF-κB dimers are largely sequestered in the cytoplasm by inhibitor-κB (IκB) proteins (Fig. 1A.i). There are at least nine proteins, including the NF-κB precursor proteins p105 and p100, that display IκB activity. All IκB proteins contain ankyrin repeats that facilitate binding to NF-κB dimers. In canonical NF-κB signaling (e.g., downstream of TLRs and TNF-α), cell stimulation leads to the phosphorylation and activation of the IκB kinase (IKK) complex, composed of IKK1, IKK2, and NEMO. The activated IKK complex then phosphorylates IκB proteins, leading to their ubiquitination and subsequent proteasome-mediated degradation. NF-κB dimers freed of inhibitors are then able to translocate to the nucleus where they bind κB promoter sites and direct transcriptional activities.

Molecular programming of steady-state DCs

A consensus in the field suggests that the predominant way to induce the adaptive immune response is via DCs that have been matured with various stimuli. However, recent evidence has demonstrated that DC immaturity is not a default state, but rather represents a quiescent steady state resulting from an undefined molecular program. Studies have shown that perturbing this programmed state leads to a destabilized DC that becomes capable of inducing T cell responses *in vivo*.

Evidence for the destabilized DC state is supported by studies by Dissanayake *et al.*[7] To examine the properties of DCs that are essential to activate CD8 function *in vivo*, a strategy was developed using transfer of bone marrow–derived DCs to induce autoimmunity. *RIP-gp* transgenic mice, which express the lymphocytic choriomeningitis virus (LCMV) glycoprotein (gp) in pancreatic islet β cells under the control of the rat insulin promoter (RIP), were vaccinated with bone marrow–derived DCs that were pulsed with gp peptides that bind to class I and class II MHC. DCs matured with TLR ligands, such as CpG DNA, induced the expansion of gp-specific T cells that were previously in a naive state. The

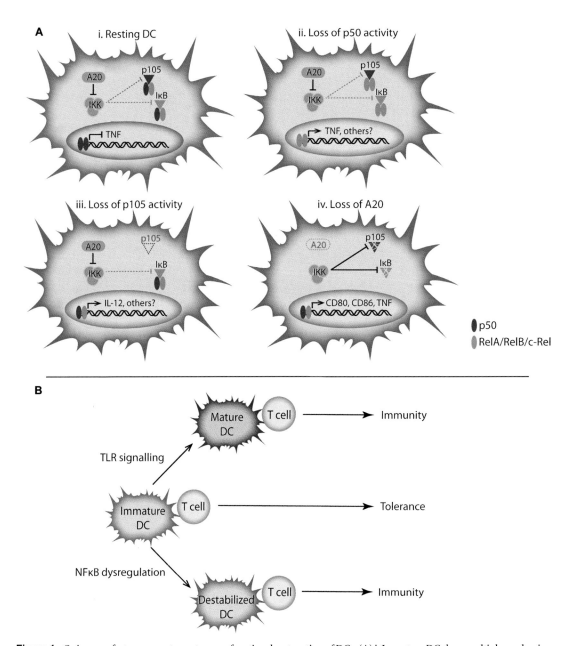

Figure 1. Quiescence factors prevent spontaneous functional maturation of DCs. (A) i. Immature DCs have multiple mechanisms to prevent aberrant maturation. A20 targets multiple proteins (RIP1, TRAFs) preventing activation of the IKK complex and release of NF-κB dimers that are sequestered in the cytoplasm by classical IκB proteins (IκBα, IκBβ, IκBε) as well as alternative IκB proteins such as p105. NF-κB p50 homodimers may bind to DNA, preventing occupancy by other activating NF-κB dimers as well as recruiting histone deacetylases, thereby blocking transcription of NF-κB target genes. ii. Loss of p50 results in liberated κB binding sites that can be bound by activating NF-κB dimers, driving transcription of genes such as TNF-α that increase DC immunogenicity. iii. Loss of p105 may result in increased NF-κB dimer nuclear localization and DNA binding, promoting the transcription of genes such as IL-12. iv. Loss of A20 results in the IKK-mediated destruction of IκB proteins, releasing them to drive expression of CD80, CD86, CD40, and TNF-α, resulting in DC maturation. (B) Normal DC homeostasis promotes immune tolerance. While immature DCs promote tolerogenic T cell responses (e.g., death, anergy, T$_{reg}$ cell induction), DCs activated through PAMP receptors such as TLRs are immunogenic and can initiate immunity. DCs that have dysregulated NF-κB signaling may become immunogenic even in the absence of exogenous stimuli. These destabilized DCs may go on to promote T cell responses against antigens derived from either healthy tissue or tumor.

generation of anti-gp immunity led to the CD8$^+$ T cell–mediated destruction of gp$^+$ pancreatic cells and, consequently, to the development of diabetes.[5,6] By contrast, immature DCs did not induce loss of tolerance. This model provides a functional readout of *in vivo* DC immunogenicity.

While NF-κB activation is widely recognized as an important component of DC activation, the individual role of each NF-κB protein in DC maturation has yet to be carefully explored. To elucidate the role of NF-κB1 in regulating DC function, the ability of NF-κB1–deficient (*Nfkb1*$^{-/-}$) bone marrow–derived DCs to induce diabetes in the *RIP-gp* model was tested; unexpectedly, in contrast with wild-type DCs, DCs lacking NF-κB1 induced diabetes in the absence of CpG stimulation.[7] These data indicate that NF-κB1 is required to maintain DCs in a quiescent state; in the absence of NF-κB1, DCs become functionally capable, in the absence of stimulation, of activating CD8$^+$ T cells *in vivo*. Immature DCs do not simply exist in a passive state; rather, factors are required to actively program DCs to remain in a resting state. The loss of NF-κB1 disrupts this homeostasis and results in DCs that are capable of breaking tolerance and inducing tissue destruction *in vivo*. Additional work showed that the functional maturation of unstimulated *Nfkb1*$^{-/-}$ DCs is associated with increased production of TNF, compared with wild-type DCs, and that TNF was required for the ability of *Nfkb1*$^{-/-}$ DCs to induce diabetes in *RIP-gp* mice. We also found that the nonquiescent *Nfkb1*$^{-/-}$ DCs do not express elevated levels of MHCII, CD80, or CD86, which suggests that upregulation of these molecules is not essential for their immunogenicity. Despite the ability of NF-κB1–deficient DCs to induce CD8$^+$ T cell responses *in vivo*, *Nfkb1*$^{-/-}$ mice do not spontaneously develop autoimmune disease, which may be due to loss of NF-κB1 in other immune populations such as T cells.

Potential role of NF-κB1 in DC homeostasis

The loss of NF-κB1 may affect DC immunogenicity through several potential mechanisms. For example, in normal DCs, p50 homodimers may maintain their resting state through transcriptional repression (Fig. 1A.ii) by competing with activating dimers for occupation of κB promoter sites and through the recruitment of histone deacetylases.[8]

This mechanism may explain why unstimulated *Nfkb1*$^{-/-}$ DCs express TNF-α, a known target of NF-κB; other genes whose products promote DC immunogenicity and may be repressed by p50 homodimers have not been identified. Alternatively, p50-containing NF-κB dimers may promote transcription of other factors that help maintain DC immaturity. For example, NF-κB dimers that lack transactivation domains, as is the case with p50 homodimers, can still promote transcription of target genes through recruitment of the adaptor molecule Bcl-3.[8]

In addition, the precursor protein p105 may be critical for maintaining DC immaturity (Fig. 1A.iii). Like other IκB proteins, p105 contains ankyrin repeats that allow it to bind to NF-κB dimers, sequestering them away from their nuclear targets. Thus, p105 may be important for repressing NF-κB binding and transactivation of genes that promote DC maturation. Consistent with this, mice deficient in p105 but not p50 suffer from chronic inflammation, demonstrating an important role of p105 in maintaining immune tolerance.[9,10] However, a direct contribution of p105 in regulating DC homeostasis has not been demonstrated, although p105 is known to regulate IL-12 in macrophages,[11] suggesting that it may play a similar role in DCs. Elucidating the mechanisms by which the NF-κB1 proteins control DC maturation will be important for the design of immunotherapies aiming to promote DC immunogenicity.

A20 programs steady-state DCs

Recent reports have identified the ubiquitin-editing enzyme A20 as another molecular checkpoint important for maintaining steady-state DCs (Fig. 1A.iv). Studies have shown that ubiquitination plays a key role in regulating NF-κB signaling pathways.[12] For example, K48-linked polyubiquitination, which induces proteosomal degradation, can either promote or inhibit NF-κB signaling by targeting either negative or positive NF-κB regulators. By contrast, K63-linked polyubiquitination of NF-κB signaling intermediates promotes signal transduction. A20 is a ubiquitin-editing enzyme that catalyzes both the hydrolysis of K63-linked polyubiquitin chains and the addition of K48-linked chains, thereby terminating signal transduction and inducing degradation of target proteins. A20 promotes K48-polyubiquitination and degradation of RIP1, a protein required for TNF-α-induced NF-κB activation, which potently inhibits NF-κB signaling. A20 can also antagonize NF-κB signaling downstream of various PAMP receptors by targeting signaling intermediates, including various TNF-α receptor–associated factor (TRAF) molecules.

Dendritic cells lacking A20 have increased NF-κB signaling and spontaneously adopt a mature phenotype, including elevated expression of CD40, CD80, CD86, MHC class II, and IL-6;[13,14] such spontaneous DC activation abolishes their ability to maintain immune tolerance. Additionally, A20-deficient DCs are hyperresponsive to stimulation with PAMPs, which leads to elevated expression of inflammatory cytokines. Mice lacking A20 specifically in DCs are predisposed to the development of autoimmune disease; one report found that A20 conditional KO mice develop systemic autoimmune disease, including the generation of anti-dsDNA autoantibodies.[14] In contrast, another report found that autoimmunity in A20 conditional knockout mice was limited to colitis and ankylosing arthritis, and did not involve autoantibody formation.[13] However, both studies detected an accumulation of activated T cells, suggesting that DC-derived A20 is essential for maintaining T cell homeostasis and tolerance. In other work, polymorphisms in A20 have been linked to the development of various autoimmune diseases, including Crohn's disease, rheumatoid arthritis, and systemic lupus erythematous. However, as A20 is a critical regulator of NF-κB in other leukocyte populations, it remains unclear in which cell population(s) these polymorphisms are driving autoimmunity.

Together, these findings demonstrate that A20 is an essential factor for the maintenance of DC immaturity and therefore critical for the preservation of immune tolerance.

Destabilized DCs, autoimmunity, and immune surveillance

Susceptibility loci for autoimmunity may include alterations in genes that maintain steady-state DCs. It is possible that individuals with changes in molecules that are important in programming immature DCs may have a hyperactive immune response that results in autoimmunity (Fig. 1B). A polymorphism has been identified in the TNF-α promoter that confers susceptibility to various autoimmune diseases;[15,16] the polymorphism has been reported to inhibit the binding of p50 homodimers to the TNF-α promoter and consequently dysregulate TNF-α production. A consequence of this polymorphism may be the development of destabilized DCs that initiate autoimmune responses. However, it remains to be seen how this polymorphism relates to autoimmune disease, and what role altered DC homeostasis may play. Likewise, as indicated previously, the A20 polymorphisms associated with autoimmune disease may affect the stabilization of immature DCs. An intriguing possibility is that patients with A20 or TNF-α promoter polymorphisms may be good candidates for cancer immune therapy since, with more easily activated DCs, they may be capable of mounting more robust immune responses against tumors. By identifying polymorphisms that control DC immunogenicity, it may be possible to define patients who have naturally stronger responses to tumor antigens. Again, such patients may be good candidates for immune modulating anticancer therapies.

The goal of cancer immunotherapy is the generation of potent antitumor immune responses. To this end, various DC-based strategies are under investigation. Although many DC vaccine-based approaches are successful in generating signs of antitumor immunity, clinical outcomes have been more limited.[17] One goal of present and future studies is to improve DC immunogenicity. Currently, functional maturation of ex vivo–generated DCs is often achieved by stimulation with cocktails comprising TNF-α, IL-6, IL-1β, and other cytokines, while other strategies use TLR ligands. However, the use of DC maturation stimuli is limited for treating patients because the materials used are not generated under appropriate manufacturing protocols considered safe for patients. A possible strategy to improve DC immunogenicity without this drawback is to target DC quiescence factors. One study showed, for example, that vaccination with NF-κB1-deficient DCs was more effective in suppressing growth of B16 melanoma than was vaccination with wild-type DCs.[18] The impact of DC quiescence factors on improving antitumor immunity warrants further examination.

Finally, understanding how DC immunogenicity is programmed, through identification of the critical molecules and pathways, will be important for the design of antitumor immunotherapies.

Acknowledgment

We would like to thank Sarah Hamilton for her critical review of the manuscript. P.S.O. holds a Canada Research Chair in Autoimmunity and Tumor Immunity.

Conflicts of interest

The authors declare no conflicts of interest.

References

1. Manicassamy, S. & B. Pulendran. 2011. Dendritic cell control of tolerogenic responses. *Immunol. Rev.* **241:** 206–227.
2. Steinman, R.M. 2012. Decisions about dendritic cells: past, present, and future. *Annu. Rev. Immunol.* **30:** 1–22.
3. Hoffmann, A. & D. Baltimore. 2006. Circuitry of nuclear factor kappaB signaling. *Immunol. Rev.* **210:** 171–186.
4. Shih, V.F. *et al.* 2012. Control of RelB during dendritic cell activation integrates canonical and noncanonical NF-kappaB pathways. *Nat. Immunol.* **13:** 1162–1170.
5. Lin, A.C. *et al.* 2011. Different toll-like receptor stimuli have a profound impact on cytokines required to break tolerance and induce autoimmunity. *PLoS One* **6:** e23940.
6. Lin, A. *et al.* 2013. ARIH2 is essential for embryogenesis, and its hematopoietic deficiency causes lethal activation of the immune system. *Nat. Immunol.* **14:** 27–33.
7. Dissanayake, D. *et al.* 2011. Nuclear factor-kappaB1 controls the functional maturation of dendritic cells and prevents the activation of autoreactive T cells. *Nat. Med.* **17:** 1663–1667.
8. Pereira, S.G. & F. Oakley. 2008. Nuclear factor-kappaB1: regulation and function. *Int. J. Biochem. Cell. Biol.* **40:** 1425–1430.
9. Ishikawa, H. *et al.* 1998. Chronic inflammation and susceptibility to bacterial infections in mice lacking the polypeptide (p)105 precursor (NF-kappaB1) but expressing p50. *J. Exp. Med.* **187:** 985–996.
10. Chang, M. *et al.* 2009. NF-kappa B1 p105 regulates T cell homeostasis and prevents chronic inflammation. *J. Immunol.* **182:** 3131–3138.
11. Zhao, X. *et al.* 2012. Nfkb1 inhibits LPS-induced IFN-beta and IL-12 p40 production in macrophages by distinct mechanisms. *PLoS One* **7:** e32811.
12. Harhaj, E.W. & V.M. Dixit. 2012. Regulation of NF-kappaB by deubiquitinases. *Immunol. Rev.* **246:** 107–124.
13. Hammer, G.E. *et al.* 2011. Expression of A20 by dendritic cells preserves immune homeostasis and prevents colitis and spondyloarthritis. *Nat. Immunol.* **12:** 1184–1193.
14. Kool, M. *et al.* 2011. The ubiquitin-editing protein A20 prevents dendritic cell activation, recognition of apoptotic cells, and systemic autoimmunity. *Immunity* **35:** 82–96.
15. Udalova, I.A. *et al.* 2000. Functional consequences of a polymorphism affecting NF-kappaB p50-p50 binding to the TNF promoter region. *Mol. Cell Biol.* **20:** 9113–9119.
16. Li, N. *et al.* 2008. Association of tumour necrosis factor alpha (TNF-alpha) polymorphisms with Graves' disease: a meta-analysis. *Clin. Biochem.* **41:** 881–886.
17. Palucka, K. & J. Banchereau. 2012. Cancer immunotherapy via dendritic cells. *Nat. Rev. Cancer* **12:** 265–277.
18. Larghi, P. *et al.* 2012. The p50 subunit of NF-kappaB orchestrates dendritic cell lifespan and activation of adaptive immunity. *PLoS One* **7:** e45279.

Ann. N.Y. Acad. Sci. ISSN 0077-8923

ANNALS OF THE NEW YORK ACADEMY OF SCIENCES

Issue: *The Renaissance of Cancer Immunotherapy*

Preventing cancer by targeting abnormally expressed self-antigens: MUC1 vaccines for prevention of epithelial adenocarcinomas

Pamela L. Beatty and Olivera J. Finn

Department of Immunology, University of Pittsburgh School of Medicine, Pittsburgh, Pennsylvania

Address for correspondence: Olivera J. Finn, University of Pittsburgh School of Medicine, E1040 Biological Sciences Tower, Pittsburgh, PA 15261. ojfinn@pitt.edu

Prophylactic vaccines based on tumor-associated antigens (TAAs) have elicited concerns due to their potential toxicity. Because TAAs are considered self-antigens, the prediction is that such vaccines will induce autoimmunity. While this has been observed in melanoma, where an antitumor immune response leads to vitiligo, autoimmunity has almost never been seen following vaccination with numerous other TAAs. We hypothesized that antigen choice determines outcome and have been working to identify TAAs whose expression differs between normal and tumor tissue, and thus could elicit antitumor immunity without autoimmunity. Studies on the epithelial TAA MUC1 have revealed that, compared to MUC1 on normal cells, tumors, premalignant lesions, and noncancerous pathologies affecting epithelial cells express abnormal MUC1, which is not a self-antigen but rather an abnormal disease-associated antigen (DAA). This distinction, which can be made for many known TAAs, has broad implications for the design and acceptance of preventative cancer vaccines.

Keywords: MUC1; immunosurveillance; tumor immunology; tumor antigens; cancer vaccines

Introduction

Therapeutic vaccines aimed to boost antitumor immune responses in cancer patients have been in clinical trials for decades, but their ability to change the course of established disease has been disappointing. The main lesson learned from these trials is that tumor microenvironments are characterized by various levels of immune suppression carried out by tumor-induced or standard therapy–induced suppressor mechanisms that weaken a patient's ability to respond either to the tumor or the vaccine. An approach that has yet to be taken is application of certain vaccines to prevention of cancer in individuals at high risk of developing disease. A way to foster such application of vaccines would be to refocus some of the attention of tumor immunologists and immunotherapists away from treating advanced and retractable cancer to treating early precursor lesions or premalignant diseases, where the potential for immune suppression and immune evasion is expected to be markedly lower.

The U.S. Food and Drug Administration's (FDA) approval and wide clinical application of vaccines against hepatitis B virus (HBV) and human papillomavirus (HPV), whose goal is to prevent cancers caused by these viruses (hepatocellular carcinoma and cervical cancer, respectively), have focused increased attention on cancer immunoprevention. These vaccines are based on target viral antigens that are expressed both during HBV and HPV infection and on cells malignantly transformed by these viruses. By inducing neutralizing antibodies to prevent the primary infection, vaccines against these antigens reduce the incidence of subsequent liver and cervical cancers. The success of these vaccines has shown that immunoprevention of cancer is possible for virally induced cancers. Unfortunately, human cancers confirmed to be caused by viruses represent less than 20% of all cancers,[1] which highlights the need to develop vaccines for prevention of nonviral cancers.

Efforts to discover tumor antigens expressed by nonviral cancers have resulted in the

doi: 10.1111/nyas.12108

identification of numerous tumor-associated antigens (TAAs) that might be candidates for such vaccines. These antigens are self-molecules expressed by normal healthy cells but become tumor antigens as a result of mutations, overexpression, or changes in posttranslational modification in tumor cells.[2] The immune system recognizes these differences and generates innate and adaptive effector mechanisms that target tumor cells that express these aberrant molecules. And while tumor-specific immune responses can be found in cancer patients, they are often within tumor-promoting microenvironments, such as those with infiltrations of myeloid-derived suppressor cells (MDSCs) in which immune responses are unable to arrest tumor growth.

Efforts to use vaccines based on TAAs in a truly preventative setting (i.e., to induce immunity against these molecules in healthy individuals at high risk for developing cancer) have met with much opposition. Because many TAAs are considered self-antigens in spite of the documented differences in expression in normal and tumor cells, the possible undesired induction of autoimmunity, in addition to useful antitumor immunity, remains the greatest theoretical concern and a barrier to testing the protective potential of these vaccines.

To date, the majority of anticancer vaccines based on TAAs have been tested in patients with advanced disease and resulted in little clinical benefit. These disappointing clinical results are not surprising, and have recently been better understood, as evidence accumulates, that the immune system has a protective role against tumors, but that it also shapes the immunogenicity of the tumor through a process of cancer immunoediting.[3] The cancer immunoediting hypothesis describes three distinct phases in tumor progression: elimination, equilibrium, and escape. Innate and adaptive immune systems work together to detect early aberrant cells in the elimination phase and prevent tumor formation. If elimination is incomplete, the remaining aberrant cells can enter an equilibrium phase during which the adaptive immune system continues to control their growth, but under increasing immune pressure. At some point, this balance is lost and cell variants can arise, leading to the escape phase exemplified by progressively growing tumors and clinical disease, and by numerous mechanisms that inhibit effective antitumor immune responses and facilitate tumor growth. The current understanding of this process

suggests that if a vaccine is administered prior to cancer occurrence, the elimination or equilibrium phase (i.e., premalignant disease) will be a more likely outcome, and escape might be prevented. For several important cancers (e.g., colon, pancreas, multiple myeloma, and melanoma) premalignant conditions have been characterized, and many of the TAAs found on the resulting tumors already begin to be expressed in the premalignant state. Animal models have shown that immune memory for these antigens induced by vaccination prior to the appearance of premalignant lesions can prevent their appearance or their progression to cancer.[4,5] Translating this to the human situation suggests that application of the vaccine in the setting of premalignant lesions could eliminate them, prevent other lesions from developing, or significantly slow their progression to cancer.

Human mucin 1 (MUC1), a large glycoprotein expressed on the apical surface of healthy ductal epithelial cells, is a well-defined TAA that has been studied as a target for immunotherapy for over a decade. Recently, MUC1 has emerged as an especially attractive target for cancer prevention based on observations that abnormal expression and glycosylation of MUC1 can be found on premalignant lesions that later become various epithelial tumors (colon, pancreas, and cervix) and nonmalignant conditions, such as transient infections or chronic inflammations (inflammatory bowel disease and endometriosis).

Here, we briefly discuss current work that characterizes abnormally expressed MUC1 as a disease-associated antigen (DAA) and a TAA rather than a self-antigen, and the importance of this distinction. We also discuss recent efforts to test the feasibility of MUC1 vaccine for cancer immunoprevention in the clinic.

Immunobiology of MUC1

A predominant characteristic of MUC1 is the variable number of tandem repeats (VNTR) region in its extracellular domain.[6] The VNTR region is comprised of a 20-amino acid sequence (PDTRPAPGSTAPPAHGVTSA) that repeats an average 20–150 times. In healthy epithelia, the VNTR is highly glycosylated on serines and threonines with long and branched O-linked carbohydrates. In the majority of adenocarcinomas, such as those of the breast, pancreas, ovary, colon and lung, and in

normal epithelium   aberrant cells   hyperplasia and dysplasia   cancer

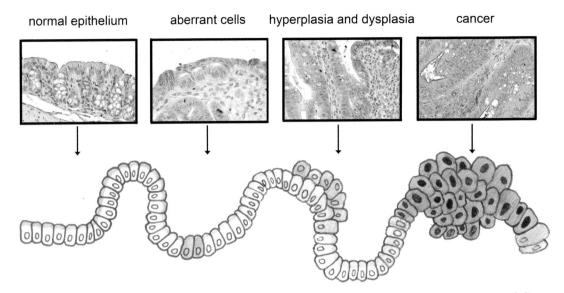

Figure 1. Changes of MUC1 expression from normal to abnormal coincide with progression from normal colonic epithelium to colon cancer. Normal MUC1 is expressed at low levels and strictly polarized to the apical surface of healthy colonic epithelial cells. Increased expression, loss of polarization, and underglycosylation of MUC1 can be detected in a few aberrant, but nonmalignant, cells present at sites of acute inflammation. Abnormal MUC1 expression further increases in hyperplasia and dysplasia (e.g., colon polyps). The highest expression of abnormal MUC1 and complete loss of polarity is found on the fully transformed colon cancer cells.

premalignant lesions leading to these cancers, MUC1 loses its apical polarization and becomes overexpressed and hypoglycosylated (Fig. 1).

This abnormal form of MUC1 is immunogenic, as the reduced glycosylation exposes the peptide backbone. Cytotoxic T lymphocytes (CTLs) specific for epitopes on the peptide backbone have been found in pancreatic,[7] breast,[8] and ovarian[9] cancer patients. Importantly, both peptide epitopes, as well as novel truncated glycopeptide epitopes from the VNTR region, can be processed and presented to the immune system to induce major histocompatibility complex (MHC)-restricted MUC1-specific CTLs.[10] MUC1-specific antibodies have been found in cancer patients and are associated with a survival benefit in breast,[11] pancreatic,[12] and ovarian[13] cancer patients.

Abnormal MUC1 expression in nonmalignant conditions

While studying MUC1 immune responses in cancer patients, we observed that these responses can also be found in individuals with no history of cancer. For example, a large retrospective case–control study showed that individuals who experienced certain conditions such as breast mastitis, pelvic surgery, or mumps virus infection of the salivary gland ducts had anti-MUC1 IgG antibodies that correlated with a reduced risk for ovarian cancer.[14] On the basis of this evidence, we proposed that each of these conditions is associated with epithelial injury and inflammation that would generate a temporal increase of abnormal expression of MUC1, similar to expression seen in cancer cells. Later in an individual's life, the appearance of nascent tumor cells expressing abnormal MUC1 would trigger immune memory that was induced by the initial noncancerous exposure to abnormal MUC1. This would result in quicker and more robust responses, compared to those of naive individuals, and lead to reduced cancer incidence.

Animal models are being developed to test this challenging proposal. One such model is used to examine the effect of repeated influenza virus infections on induction of anti-MUC1 immunity in MUC1 transgenic (MUC1 tg) mice and their subsequent response to a challenge with a MUC1-expressing tumor. Our work in progress has found overexpression and abnormal glycosylation of MUC1 in the lungs of flu-infected MUC1 tg mice, compared with control uninfected MUC1 tg mice, and MUC1-specific CD8$^+$ T cells can be detected in spleens of infected MUC1 tg mice. Eighty days after a second flu infection, mice are challenged with a MUC1-expressing tumor; thus far, the data indicate a dramatic difference in the kinetics of tumor growth, and a statistically significant difference in tumor size, between influenza-infected and naive MUC1 tg mice. These experiments are ongoing.

Abnormal MUC1 expression in chronic inflammation and premalignant disease

Overexpression and abnormal glycosylation of MUC1 has also been found in the inflamed colon of patients suffering from inflammatory bowel disease (IBD).[15] Results from MUC1 tg mouse models of human IBD showed that expression of abnormal MUC1 increased IBD pathogenesis and progression to colitis-associated colon cancer (CACC).[15] This outcome could be prevented by administration of a MUC1 vaccine early in disease, which ameliorated IBD symptoms and protected from progression to CACC. The MUC1 vaccine induced production of MUC1-specific IgG antibodies and MUC1-specific T cells that eliminated cells expressing the abnormal form of MUC1.[4,5] Importantly, no autoimmune side effects were detected in treated animals.[4]

In addition, overexpression and abnormal glycosylation of MUC1 has been observed in other chronic inflammatory conditions, such as endometriosis,[16] pancreatitis,[17] and Barrett's esophagus (BE). Besides a chronic inflammatory condition of the esophagus, BE is also the only known precursor lesion, and most important risk factor, for esophageal adenocarcinoma.[18] The mucosal injury in BE has been shown to result from gastroesophageal reflux disease (GERD), in which bile acids have been reported to induce MUC1 expression in human esophageal tissues[19] (and unpublished data, P.L. Beatty and O.J. Finn). Tumor forms of MUC1 have also been found in pancreatic intraepithelial neoplasia (PanINs), precursors of pancreatic cancer. Increased MUC1 expression correlated with the grade and severity of PanIN lesions.[20] In addition, abnormal MUC1 expression was increased on pancreatic cysts from patients as well as in mouse tumor models.[21] And MUC1 has been found to be significantly overexpressed in colonic polyps, the extent of expression and abnormal glycosylation correlating with polyp size, degree of dysplasia, and villous histology.[22–24] In addition, MUC1-specific IgG has been detected in patients with a history of adenomatous polyps (P.L. Beatty and O.J. Finn, unpublished data).

Clinical trials of MUC1 vaccines for cancer prevention

Our findings of abnormal MUC1 expression in chronic inflammation and premalignant disease prompted us to design and implement a recent completion of a phase I/II trial of a prophylactic MUC1 peptide vaccine in 40 patients with a history of advanced colon adenoma, precursors of colon cancer.[25] This was the first immunopreventive vaccine trial that used a TAA rather than a viral antigen. Importantly, this study showed that the vaccine can elicit high levels of MUC1-specific IgG antibody without significant toxicity. Individuals who did not respond to the vaccine were found to have high numbers of MDSCs prior to vaccination, indicating that immunosuppression in some individuals is already present in the premalignant setting. This suggests the utility of prophylactic vaccination at even earlier times in disease development or, ideally, in individuals without any evidence of premalignant disease but who have a known risk for colon cancer. A phase II randomized efficacy trial is being set up that will evaluate the ability of the MUC1 vaccine, and its elicited immune response, to prevent polyp recurrence, and thereby prevent new colon cancers.

Conclusions

Over the past 30 years, results from studies have revealed that abnormal MUC1 is expressed in a majority of mature tumors, in many premalignant lesions, and in noncancerous events affecting epithelial cells, such as injury, infection, and acute or chronic inflammation. As such, MUC1 TAA should be considered a DAA rather than a self-antigen. Plenty of evidence indicates that many other molecules identified as TAAs due to abnormal expression on tumors are also DAAs.[26,27] This distinction is important because it changes the current thinking about immunosurveillance of cancer and infections as being mutually exclusive events: our studies show, in fact, that targets of antitumor and antipathogen immune responses can be the same. The current data on MUC1 are summarized previously; hopefully, future studies will provide information on additional TAAs expressed in infections and other diseases.

Eliciting immune memory through vaccination against one or more of these targets may have a more general protective function than that provided by current vaccines directed against specific pathogens or cancers.

Conflicts of interest

The authors declare no conflicts of interest.

References

1. Thun, M.J. *et al.* 2010. The global burden of cancer: priorities for prevention. *Carcinogenesis* **31:** 100–110.

2. Finn, O.J. 2008. Cancer immunology. *N. Engl. J. Med.* **358:** 2704–2715.

3. Schreiber, R.D., L.J. Old & M.J. Smyth. 2011. Cancer immunoediting: integrating immunity's roles in cancer suppression and promotion. *Science* **331:** 1565–1570.

4. Beatty, P., S. Ranganathan & O.J. Finn 2012. Prevention of colitis-associated colon cancer using a vaccine to target abnormal expression of the MUC1 tumor antigen. *Oncoimmunology* **1:** 263–270.

5. Beatty, P.L. *et al.* 2010. Vaccine against MUC1 antigen expressed in inflammatory bowel disease and cancer lessens colonic inflammation and prevents progression to colitis-associated colon cancer. *Cancer Prev. Res.* **3:** 438–446.

6. Vlad, A.M. *et al.* 2004. MUC1 immunobiology: from discovery to clinical applications. *Adv. Immunol.* **82:** 249–293.

7. Barnd, D.L. *et al.* 1989. Specific, major histocompatibility complex-unrestricted recognition of tumor-associated mucins by human cytotoxic T cells. *Proc. Natl. Acad. Sci. USA* **86:** 7159–7163.

8. Jerome, K.R. *et al.* 1991. Cytotoxic T-lymphocytes derived from patients with breast adenocarcinoma recognize an epitope present on the protein core of a mucin molecule preferentially expressed by malignant cells. *Cancer Res.* **51:** 2908–2916.

9. Ioannides, C.G. *et al.* 1993. Cytotoxic T cells from ovarian malignant tumors can recognize polymorphic epithelial mucin core peptides. *J. Immunol.* **151:** 3693–3703.

10. Vlad, A.M. *et al.* 2002. Complex carbohydrates are not removed during processing of glycoproteins by dendritic cells: processing of tumor antigen MUC1 glycopeptides for presentation to major histocompatibility complex class II-restricted T cells. *J. Exp. Med.* **196:** 1435–1446.

11. von Mensdorff-Pouilly, S. *et al.* 2000. Survival in early breast cancer patients is favorably influenced by a natural humoral immune response to polymorphic epithelial mucin. *J. Clin. Oncol.* **18:** 574–583.

12. Hamanaka, Y. *et al.* 2003. Circulating anti-MUC1 IgG antibodies as a favorable prognostic factor for pancreatic cancer. *Int. J. Cancer.* **103:** 97–100.

13. Pinheiro, S.P. *et al.* Anti-MUC1 antibodies and ovarian cancer risk: prospective data from the Nurses' Health Studies. *Cancer Epidemiol. Biomarkers Prev.* **19:** 1595–1601.

14. Cramer, D.W. *et al.* 2005. Conditions associated with antibodies against the tumor-associated antigen MUC1 and their relationship to risk for ovarian cancer. *Cancer Epidemiol. Biomarkers Prev.* **14:** 1125–1131.

15. Beatty, P.L. *et al.* 2007. Cutting edge: transgenic expression of human MUC1 in IL-10$^{-/-}$ mice accelerates inflammatory bowel disease and progression to colon cancer. *J. Immunol.* **179:** 735–739.

16. Vlad, A.M., I. Diaconu & K.R. Gantt. 2006. MUC1 in endometriosis and ovarian cancer. *Immunol. Res.* **36:** 229–236.

17. Kadayakkara, D.K. *et al.* 2010. Inflammation driven by overexpression of the hypoglycosylated abnormal mucin 1 (MUC1) links inflammatory bowel disease and pancreatitis. *Pancreas* **39:** 510–515.

18. Wiseman, E.F. & Y.S. Ang 2011. Risk factors for neoplastic progression in Barrett's esophagus. *World J. Gastroenterol.* **17:** 3672–3683.

19. Mariette, C. *et al.* 2008. Activation of MUC1 mucin expression by bile acids in human esophageal adenocarcinomatous cells and tissues is mediated by the phosphatidylinositol 3-kinase. *Surgery* **143:** 58–71.

20. Yonezawa, S. *et al.* 2008. Precursor lesions of pancreatic cancer. *Gut Liver* **2:** 137–154.

21. Finn, O.J. *et al.* 2011. Importance of MUC1 and spontaneous mouse tumor models for understanding the immunobiology of human adenocarcinomas. *Immunol. Res.* **50:** 261–268.

22. Ajioka, Y., H. Watanabe & J.R. Jass. 1997. MUC1 and MUC2 mucins in flat and polypoid colorectal adenomas. *J. Clin. Pathol.* **50:** 417–421.

23. Ho, S.B. *et al.* 1996. Altered mucin core peptide immunoreactivity in the colon polyp-carcinoma sequence. *Oncol. Res.* **8:** 53–61.

24. Zotter, S. *et al.* 1987. Immunohistochemical localization of the epithelial marker MAM-6 in invasive malignancies and highly dysplastic adenomas of the large intestine. *Lab. Invest.* **57:** 193–199.

25. Kimura, T. *et al.* 2013. MUC1 vaccine for individuals with advanced adenoma of the colon: a Cancer Immunoprevention Feasibility Study. *Cancer Prev. Res.* **6:** 18–26.

26. Savage, P.A. *et al.* 2008. Recognition of a ubiquitous self antigen by prostate cancer-infiltrating CD8$^+$ T lymphocytes. *Science* **319:** 215–220.

27. Vella, L.A. *et al.* 2009. Healthy individuals have T-cell and antibody responses to the tumor antigen cyclin B1 that when elicited in mice protect from cancer. *Proc. Natl. Acad. Sci. USA* **106:** 14010–14015.

Ann. N.Y. Acad. Sci. ISSN 0077-8923

ANNALS OF THE NEW YORK ACADEMY OF SCIENCES

Issue: *The Renaissance of Cancer Immunotherapy*

Immunological control of cell cycle aberrations for the avoidance of oncogenesis: the case of tetraploidy

Laura Senovilla,[1,2,3] Lorenzo Galluzzi,[2,5] Maria Castedo,[1,2,3,*] and Guido Kroemer[1,4,5,6,7,*]

[1]INSERM, U848, Villejuif, France. [2]Institut Gustave Roussy, Villejuif, France. [3]Université Paris Sud /Paris XI, Le Kremlin Bicêtre, France. [4]Université Paris Descartes/Paris, France. [5]Centre de Recherche des Cordeliers, Paris, France. [6]Metabolomics Platform, Institut Gustave Roussy, Villejuif, France. [7]Pôle de Biologie, Hôpital Européen Georges Pompidou, AP-HP, Paris, France

Address for correspondence: Guido Kroemer, M.D., Ph.D., INSERM, U848, Institut Gustave Roussy, Pavillon de Recherche 1, 39 rue Camille Desmoulins, F-94805 Villejuif, France. kroemer@orange.fr

Tetraploid cells—cells that contain twice the normal amount of DNA—are more prone to neoplastic transformation than their normal, diploid counterparts since they are genomically unstable and frequently undergo asymmetric, multipolar cell divisions. Similar to many other genomic aberrations, tetraploidization is normally avoided by multiple, nonredundant cell-intrinsic mechanisms that are tied to cell cycle checkpoints. Unexpectedly, tetraploidization is also under the control of a cell-extrinsic mechanism determined by the immune system. Indeed, oncogene- or carcinogen-induced cancers developing in immunodeficient mice contain cells with a higher DNA content than similar tumors growing in immunocompetent hosts. Moreover, cancer cell lines that have been rendered tetraploid *in vitro* grow normally in immunodeficient mice, yet almost fail to generate tumors in immunocompetent animals. One of the mechanisms whereby the immune system recognizes tetraploid cells originates from tetraploidy causing an endoplasmic reticulum (ER) stress response that culminates in the exposure of the ER protein calreticulin on the cell surface. Hence, tetraploidy exemplifies a potentially oncogenic alteration that is repressed by a combination of cell-autonomous mechanisms and immunosurveillance. Oncogenesis and tumor progression require the simultaneous failure of both such control systems.

Keywords: calreticulin; CT26 cells; eIF2α phosphorylation; HMGB1; nocodazole; p53

Introduction

As they evolve, (pre-)malignant cells accumulate a plethora of genetic and epigenetic alterations that, at least initially, activate cell-autonomous (intrinsic) and immune system–mediated (extrinsic) oncosuppressive mechanisms. Intrinsic oncosuppression generally involves either (1) the repair of intracellular damage and/or the correction of cell cycle abnormalities, leading to the reestablishment of homeostasis, or (2) the activation of a permanent cell cycle arrest (senescence) or programmed cell death when the extent of damage is beyond recovery. In addition, potentially malignant cells can be specifically recognized and eliminated by immunosurveillance, relying on a combination of innate and cognate effector mechanisms.[1,2] Only once these intrinsic and extrinsic barriers to carcinogenesis have been infringed can malignant progression proceed unrestrained. This means that, to form a macroscopic neoplasm, (pre-)malignant cells must (i) inactivate the cell-autonomous checkpoint mechanisms that would normally lead to their senescence or death, and (ii) avoid immune recognition, either by passively losing the properties that render them immunogenic (a process that is referred to as *immunoselection* or *immunoediting*) or by actively suppressing immune responses (a process that is referred to as *immunosubversion*). Hence, clinically manifest cancers proceed from an initial phase in which (pre-)malignant cells are actively eliminated,

---

*Share senior co-authorship.

doi: 10.1111/nyas.12072

Ann. N.Y. Acad. Sci. 1284 (2013) 57–61 © 2013 New York Academy of Sciences.

through an equilibrium state in which smoldering neoplastic lesions are kept under control by the immune system, to a final step of complete escape from immunosurveillance.[1]

Patients are generally diagnosed with cancer when lesions are macroscopically detectable, most often when neoplastic cells have already invaded local tissues or metastasized to distant sites, implying that they have efficiently subverted immunosurveillance. During the last decade, it has become increasingly clear that the long-term success of conventional and experimental anticancer therapies often, if not always, relies on the induction of anticancer immune responses that reactivate immunosurveillance.[3] One of the mechanisms that operate in this sense is immunogenic cell death (ICD), a functionally peculiar type of apoptosis that can be elicited by some, but not all, therapeutic regimens. ICD *de facto* converts the patient's dying malignant cells into a therapeutic vaccine, hence stimulating a tumor-specific immune response that, at least in some circumstances, can control (and sometimes even eradicate) residual cancer cells.[4] What are the clinical and experimental arguments in support of the possible contribution of an anticancer immune response elicited by dying tumor cells to the success of chemotherapy?

First, the meta-analysis of multiple clinical studies indicates that severe lymphopenia ($<1,000$ cells/μL) negatively affects the chemotherapeutic response of distinct solid neoplasms. Accordingly, a collection of murine cancers (including transplantable tumors as well as chemically-induced, primary cancers) respond to chemotherapy with ICD inducers (e.g., anthracyclines or oxaliplatin) much more efficiently when they develop in syngenic immunocompetent mice than in immunodeficient hosts. Anthracycline-killed tumor cells appear to be particularly immunogenic also in humans, and have already been used with success for the therapeutic vaccination of cancer patients.[3]

Second, the composition, function, and gene expression profile of the intratumoral immune infiltrate have been shown to critically influence disease outcome in dozens, if not hundreds, of cancer patient cohorts. In particular, tumor infiltration by interferon γ (IFN-γ)–producing CD8[+] memory effector T cells has been ascribed with a consistent prognostic value and, at least in some clinical settings (e.g., breast carcinoma patients un-

dergoing neoadjuvant chemotherapy), with a predictive potential. Thus, an increased ratio of cytotoxic CD8[+] T cells over FOXP3[+] regulatory T cells postchemotherapy reportedly predicts favorable therapeutic responses in human breast and colorectal cancer.[3,5]

Third, chemotherapy-elicited immune responses obligatorily rely on dendritic cells (DCs), which engulf, process, and present antigens from dying tumor cells, as well as on several subpopulations of T lymphocytes, including, but not limited to, IFN-γ– secreting CD8[+] and interleukin (IL)-17–producing Th17 CD4[+] cells. In mice, DCs perceive the death of cancer cells as immunogenic, thanks to Toll-like receptor 4 (TLR4) and the purinergic receptor P2rx7. In line with this notion, loss-of-function mutations in *Tlr4* and *P2RX7* constitute negative predictors of the clinical response to adjuvant chemotherapy with anthracyclines or oxaliplatin in breast cancer patients.[3]

Based on these premises, we believe that anticancer therapy–elicited ICD has a major clinical impact. As an operational definition, we propose that ICD should fulfill the following two criteria. First, cells that undergo ICD *in vitro* and are injected into mice should protect them against a subsequent challenge with live tumor cells of the same kind. Second, the induction of ICD *in vivo* should provoke a local response featuring the influx of immune effector cells into the tumor parenchyma, and hence mediate antitumor effects that depend, at least in part, on the immune system.[4]

It should be noted that most cytotoxic agents fail to elicit ICD, with the notable exceptions of anthracyclines, oxaliplatin, cyclophosphamide, and cardiac glycosides.[4,6] Of note, even structurally similar chemicals, such as oxaliplatin and cisplatin, may not be equivalent in their capacity to induce ICD, implying that there is no simple structure–function relationship in this respect. Rather, the capacity of a given intervention to elicit ICD must be assessed either *in vivo* (as described previously, representing the gold standard approach) or *in vitro*, based on three surrogate markers of ICD: the early exposure of calreticulin (CRT) on the cell surface, the active secretion of ATP during the blebbing phase of apoptosis, and the release of the nonhistone chromatin-binding protein high mobility group box 1 (HMGB1) upon the permeabilization of both the nuclear and the plasma membrane.[4]

Identification of ICD inducers

In an attempt to identify novel inducers of ICD, we performed a chemical screen and found that several agents, including taxanes, epothilones, and cytochalasins, stimulated the exposure of CRT on the surface while promoting tetraploidization (the acquisition of two copies of the genome), owing to their capacity to inhibit the microtubule-dependent division of nuclei (i.e., karyokinesis) or the actin cytoskeleton–dependent division of cellular bodies (i.e., cytokinesis).[7] Subsequent functional analyses revealed that the exposure of CRT in response to tetraploidizing agents does not depend on the initiating stimulus, but rather stems from the tetraploidization process itself. Indeed, all cell types investigated were found to react to tetraploidization by activating an endoplasmic reticulum (ER) stress response that (1) is required for the survival of tetraploid cells, and (2) leads to the constitutive exposure of CRT (which is usually confined in the ER lumen) on the cell surface. Moreover, dying tetraploid cells inoculated into immunocompetent mice elicited protective anticancer immune responses in vaccination experiments.[7]

Of note, tetraploidy can arise via several distinct mechanisms, including the illicit fusion of two somatic cells, two subsequent rounds of DNA replication (S phases) in the absence of an intervening mitosis (endoreplication), or an abortive mitosis that fails either before anaphase or at cytokinesis (endomitosis). Tetraploid cells constitute stochastic generators of genomic instability because they are prone to lose chromosomes during subsequent rounds of abnormal, but bipolar, mitoses (generating two daughter cells) or even undergo asymmetric multipolar mitoses (generating three or more daughter cells). Such events contribute to pleomorphy, that is, an elevated degree of heterogeneity in cellular/nuclear size and shape. Pleomorphy is commonly viewed as a sign of malignancy, often correlating with high tumor grade and increased aggressiveness.[8]

To gain further insights into the relationship between tetraploidy and tumor immunosurveillance, we used a variety of experimental approaches. Thus, we generated stably near-to-tetraploid (hereafter referred to as hyperploid) clones from near-to-diploid (hereafter referred to as pseudodiploid) murine cancer cells, including CT26 colorectal carcinoma, Lewis lung carcinomas, and MCA205 fibrosarcoma cells, by transiently exposing them to nocodazole (a reversible microtubule inhibitor) followed by cytofluorometric purification. Such hyperploid cells grew normally *in vitro* and *in vivo* in severely immunodeficient mice lacking both the Rag2 recombinase (which is required for the productive recombination of genes coding for immunoglobulins and T cell receptors) and the common cytokine receptor γ chain (which is necessary for the development of all types of lymphocytes including B, T, NK, and NKT cells). Conversely, hyperploid cells often failed to generate tumors when injected under the skin of histocompatible immunocompetent mice in the same conditions in which their pseudodiploid progenitors efficiently did so.[7] In a reduced proportion of cases, hyperploid cells eventually formed palpable tumors even in immunocompetent mice, although such lesions became apparent only after a considerable latency. Strikingly, the malignant cells that could be recovered from immunoselected tumors (i.e., arising from hyperploid cells implanted into immunocompetent mice) exhibited a significant reduction in DNA content and chromosomal number as compared to those isolated from tumors formed by hyperploid cells in immunodeficient mice. Hence, the immune system appears to counterselect the growth of cells with an increased ploidy. Subsequent mechanistic studies revealed that the correlation between tetraploidy, ER stress, and CRT exposure is maintained *in vivo*. Immunoselection led indeed to the preferential elimination of cells manifesting a triad of (1) elevated chromosome content, (2) signs of ER stress, and (3) the translocation of CRT to the outer leaflet of the plasma membrane. Experiments in which CRT was artificially depleted (by means of small-interfering RNAs) or tethered to the plasma membrane (upon the transgene-driven expression of a genetically engineered CRT variant) confirmed the importance of CRT for immunoselection. On one hand, the depletion of CRT from hyperploid cells rendered them capable of growing unhampered in immunocompetent mice. On the other hand, the enforced expression of membrane-bound CRT reduced the growth of pseudodiploid cancer cells in immunocompetent, but not immunodeficient, mice. Thus, pseudodiploid cells constitutively exposing CRT on their surface generated palpable lesions only once they

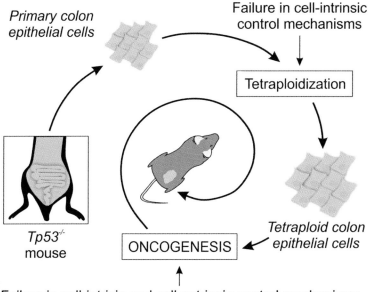

Figure 1. An immunosurveillance mechanism that avoids oncogenesis as driven by tetraploid primary epithelial cells. Colonocytes obtained from $Tp53^{-/-}$ (but not from wild-type) mice are susceptible to both spontaneous and drug-induced tetraploidization *in vitro*, implying that they lack essential cell-intrinsic control mechanisms that normally ensure the maintenance of diploidy. In syngenic immunocompetent animals, tetraploid $Tp53^{-/-}$ colon crypt organoids—whose cells exhibit increased baseline levels of endoplasmic reticulum stress and surface exposure of the immunogenic protein calreticulin—are unable to efficiently form tumors. Conversely, the growth of tetraploid $Tp53^{-/-}$ colon crypt organoids proceeds unrestrained in immunodeficient mice. These observations point to the existence of an immunosurveillance mechanism that (pre-)malignant tetraploid cells must evade for oncogenesis to progress.

had been immunoselected for the loss of membrane-bound CRT expression.[7]

In an additional series of experiments, we determined whether the tetraploidization of primary cells can drive oncogenesis (Fig. 1). To this aim, we took advantage of primary colon epithelial cells obtained from $Tp53^{-/-}$ mice (since p53 depletion is a prerequisite for the long-term survival of tetraploid cells) and rendered them tetraploid *in vitro*. Such cells were able to form normal colon crypt organoids *in vitro*, although they manifested an elevated degree of CRT exposure at the cell surface. Moreover, tetraploid colonocytes generated lesions exhibiting histopathological signs of malignancy upon the subcutaneous injection into immunodeficient $Rag2^{-/-}\gamma c^{-/-}$ (but not immunocompetent) mice.[9] These results confirm the capacity of the immune system to selectively recognize and destroy tetraploid cells.

To further explore the impact of the immune system on ploidy, we induced the development of a series of cancers (with specific chemical or genetic manipulations) in immunocompetent (wild-type) mice or in animals that were immunodeficient, either owing to the $Rag2^{-/-}\gamma c^{-/-}$ genotype or to a lack of other essential genes, such as *Stat1* or *Dnam1*. In particular, B cell lymphomas were induced by the overexpression of the *Myc* oncogene, skin fibrosarcomas by means of the chemical carcinogen methylcholanthrene, and breast carcinomas by a combination of hormonal stimulation (with medroxyprogesterone acetate) and DNA damage (with 7,12-dimethylbenz[α]anthracene). In all of these models, we found that neoplastic lesions developing in immunodeficient mice contain larger nuclei (reflecting a higher DNA content) and undergo more pronounced ER stress (as assessed by the phosphorylation status of eIF2α, a critical substrate of the ER stress–associated kinase PERK) than similar tumors growing in wild-type mice. Finally, in a cohort of breast cancer patients treated with anthracyclines (which are *bona fide* ICD inducers), we found that the infiltration of the tumor bed by cytotoxic T cells correlates positively with the elimination of cancer cells bearing large (and hence presumably hyperploid) nuclei and displaying the ER stress–associated phosphorylation of eIF2α, supporting the probable clinical relevance of our findings.[9]

Conclusions

Our work revealed the existence of an immunosurveillance mechanism that controls the ploidy of tumor cells and their precursors. At this stage, many issues remain to be elucidated. Are there acquired features of (pre-)malignant cells other than an increased ploidy[7] and the exposure of NK cell–activating ligands[10] that can elicit immunosurveillance? Which are the immune effector systems that mediate the first-line defense against hyperploidy? What are the exact mechanisms through which hyperploid cells are recognized and destroyed by the immune system? We anticipate that answers to these questions may yield important insights into the molecular and cellular circuitries underpinning natural and therapy-induced anticancer immunosurveillance.

Acknowledgments

This work is supported by grants to G.K. from the Ligue Nationale contre le Cancer (Equipe labellisée), Agence Nationale pour la Recherche (ANR), AXA Chair for Longevity Research (AXA Foundation), European Commission (ArtForce, ChemoRes), Fondation pour la Recherche Médicale (FRM), Institut National du Cancer (INCa), Cancéropôle Ile-de-France, Fondation Bettencourt-Schueller, the LabEx Immuno-Oncology, and the Paris Alliance of Cancer Research Institutes (PACRI).

Conflicts of interest

The authors declare no conflicts of interest.

References

1. Schreiber, R.D., L.J. Old & M.J. Smyth. 2011. Cancer immunoediting: integrating immunity's roles in cancer suppression and promotion. *Science* **331:** 1565–1570.
2. O'Sullivan, T. *et al.* 2012. Cancer immunoediting by the innate immune system in the absence of adaptive immunity. *J. Exp. Med.* **209:** 1869–1882.
3. Zitvogel, L., O. Kepp & G. Kroemer. 2011. Immune parameters affecting the efficacy of chemotherapeutic regimens. *Nat. Rev. Clin. Oncol.* **8:** 151–160.
4. Kroemer, G. *et al.* 2013. Immunogenic cell death in cancer therapy. *Annu. Rev. Immunol.*
5. Michaud, M. *et al.* 2011. Autophagy-dependent anticancer immune responses induced by chemotherapeutic agents in mice. *Science* **334:** 1573–1577.
6. Menger, L. *et al.* 2012. Cardiac glycosides exert anticancer effects by inducing immunogenic cell death. *Sci. Transl. Med.* **4:** 143ra199.
7. Senovilla, L. *et al.* 2012. An immunosurveillance mechanism controls cancer cell ploidy. *Science* **337:** 1678–1684.
8. Davoli, T. & T. de Lange. 2011. The causes and consequences of polyploidy in normal development and cancer. *Annu. Rev. Cell Develop. Biol.* **27:** 585–610.
9. Boileve, A., L. Senovilla, I. Vitale, *et al.* 2013. Immunosurveillance against tetraploidization-induced colon tumorigenesis. *Cell Cycle* **12:** 473–479.
10. Raulet, D.H. & N. Guerra. 2009. Oncogenic stress sensed by the immune system: role of natural killer cell receptors. *Nat. Rev. Immunol.* **9:** 568–580.

Ann. N.Y. Acad. Sci. ISSN 0077-8923

Ongoing adaptive immune responses in the microenvironment of melanoma metastases

Nicolas van Baren[1,2] and Pierre G. Coulie[2]

[1]Ludwig Institute for Cancer Research Ltd., Brussels, Belgium. [2]de Duve Institute, Université Catholique de Louvain, Brussels, Belgium

Address for correspondence: Nicolas van Baren, Ludwig Institute for Cancer Reseach Ltd., Brussels Branch, 74 Avenue Hippocrate, B1–74.03, B-1200 Brussels, Belgium. nicolas.vanbaren@bru.licr.org

A large body of evidence supports the idea that the tumor environment is immunosuppressive, notably for T lymphocytes. Yet, in some tumor types, the presence of tumor-infiltrating T cells has favorable prognostic value. In order to better understand the functional value of T cells in human tumors, we focused on cutaneous metastases of melanoma and observed that some of them host ectopic lymphoid structures in which B cell, and possibly T cell, responses take place. This observation is discussed in the context of current views on immunosuppression in tumors.

Keywords: melanoma; metastasis; lymphoid neogenesis; germinal center; humoral response; IgA

Introduction

The last two decades have seen major improvements in our understanding of immune responses directed at human malignancies. Many key findings were made on melanoma, presumably because this tumor, more than others, is able to give rise to immortalized cell lines when grown in culture, which has allowed extensive immunological investigations *in vitro*. With this model, we have learned that most, if not all, tumors carry antigens that can be targeted by T lymphocytes. These antigens, small peptides derived from endogenous proteins and bound to human leukocyte antigen (HLA) molecules, are either absent or have a restricted expression in healthy tissues.[1] Use of tumor-specific antigens in therapeutic vaccines has resulted in tumor regressions in some metastatic melanoma patients, including a few durable remissions. However, the vast majority of patients failed to display tumor responses. Among the various vaccine modalities that have been tested, no single one has emerged with clearly superior antitumoral activity.

Much effort has been devoted to the analysis of cytotoxic T cell (CTL) responses and of the tumors of selected vaccinated patients.[2] Overall, antivaccine CTL responses have been found to be either weak or undetectable, even in patients who had displayed an objective tumor regression following vaccination.[2–4] While investigating these responses, it was observed that many patients with advanced melanoma had mounted spontaneous T cell responses against some of these antigens, implying that antitumoral immunity failed to control tumor progression in these patients.[5] The failure of spontaneous and vaccine-induced immune responses is attributed to various mechanisms of either tumor resistance to immune attack or local inhibition of T cell responses.[6] Such mechanisms are presumably selected by the tumor during its progression under immune pressure. Among the many candidate mechanisms of immune suppression proposed, at least two T cell inhibitory pathways, CD28/CTLA-4 and PD-1/PD-L1, appear to play a role, because their inhibition by anti-CTLA-4, anti-PD-1, and anti-PD-L1 antibody therapies leads to clinical responses.[7,8]

These remarkable successes should not obscure our ignorance of several important parameters of human tumor immunology. While we know that tumors are antigenic and understand the molecular causes of this antigenicity, we still do not know how, when, and where antitumor T cell responses originate, are maintained and

doi: 10.1111/nyas.12093

amplified, and how they evolve during disease progression. The molecular determinants that are present in the tumor environment, activate innate immunity, and attract inflammatory cells, are largely unknown. Finally, the precise mechanisms of resistance or immune suppression that are active in human tumors remain poorly characterized. Indeed, the low proportions of patients responding to anti-CTLA4, anti-PD1, or PD-L1 antibodies suggest that alternative mechanisms play an important role.

Melanoma metastases host adaptive immune responses

Among the many candidates proposed, soluble factors (e.g., transforming growth factor beta (TGF-β), interleukin 10, galectins) or suppressive cells (e.g., regulatory T cells, myeloid-derived suppressor cells, tumor-associated macrophages, tolerogenic dendritic cells) that cause immunosuppression in the tumor environment are the most frequently cited. Numerous murine models support these candidates, even though their relevance to human malignancies remains to be demonstrated by selectively eliminating these cells or inhibiting their function. The tumor environment is thus often considered to be deeply immunosuppressed, infiltrated by anergized or exhausted lymphocytes. However, it has been shown in large tumor series that the presence of tumor-infiltrating T lymphocytes is associated with a relatively more favorable prognosis,[9] which strongly suggests that these lymphocytes, many of which display an activated phenotype, exert some antitumoral activity.

Another recent observation that challenges the view of a strong immunosuppression within tumors comes from studying the inflammatory and immune infiltrates present in cutaneous melanoma metastases. It was observed that, in some of the infiltrates, clusters of B lymphocytes centered around a network of follicular dendritic cells.[10] These structures were associated with high endothelial venule–like blood vessels and clusters of mature dendritic cells and T cells, together forming so-called ectopic or tertiary lymphoid structures (Fig. 1).[10] Some B cell follicles contained small germinal centers. Similar observations have been made in other tumor types, indicating that lymphoid neogenesis is a widespread phenomenon in human malignancies.[11–13]

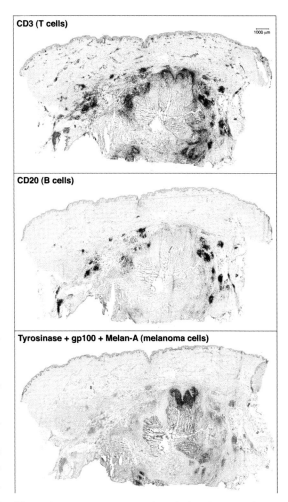

Figure 1. Microscopic images of B and T lymphocytes infiltrating a cutaneous melanoma metastasis. Sequential cryosections from tumor LB2708-MEL were immunostained against the indicated antigens and counterstained with hematoxylin. Positively stained antigens appear in red. The B cells are concentrated in follicles associated with T cell clusters. These structures correspond to ectopic lymphoid structures, similar to those previously described.[10]

The molecular analysis of rearranged immunoglobulin genes isolated from microdissected regions within melanoma lymphoid follicles indicated the occurrence of clonal B cell amplification, isotype switching, clonal diversity, and unproductive rearrangements, which are common characteristics of antibody affinity maturation. Isotype switching toward IgG1, IgG2, IgA1, and IgA2 were found,[10] and, surprisingly, IgA responses were detected, which had never been documented in ectopic lymphoid structures, let alone within tumors. The main soluble factor that participates in T-dependent IgA class switching is TGF-β, which is secreted by many cell types but usually as its inactive form latent TGF-β, a noncovalent association of TGF-β and latency-associated peptide. A possible source of active TGF-β is regulatory T cells, which are not only capable of producing latent TGF-β but also converting it into active TGF-β.[14] Interestingly, follicular regulatory T cells have been described in mice,[15, 16] and they might prevent autoantibody production following somatic hypermutation. Whether TGF-β participates in this enforcement of self-tolerance is not known.

Our results indicate that antibodies are produced locally within human melanoma metastases outside of secondary lymphoid organs. Whether these local antibody responses are directed at melanoma antigens has not yet been demonstrated. Antibodies to melanoma antigens such as tyrosinase, MAGE, or NY-ESO-1 proteins can be found in the serum of melanoma patients prior to immunotherapy, and it is possible that such antibodies are actually produced locally. B lymphocytes present in these tertiary lymphoid follicles could be an interesting source of reagents recognizing unknown melanoma antigens; this is even more interesting for other types of tumors, against which it has not been possible to derive tumor-specific T cells, owing to the absence of autologous tumor cell lines. Regarding local T cell responses, their occurrence is suggested by the association of T cells and mature dendritic cells present in ectopic lymphoid structures.

Concluding remarks

Altogether, our observations indicate that adaptive immune responses can take place inside the melanoma environment. The clinical consequences of this phenomenon are unknown. The presence of ectopic lymphoid structures in melanoma and in lung and colorectal cancer has been associated with a relatively more favorable prognosis in preliminary reports,[9, 12, 13] which, if confirmed, would suggest that these local adaptive responses contribute to tumor control. Lymphoid neogenesis is found in many chronic inflammatory diseases, where it is induced by persistent lymphocyte activation that fails to eradicate an antigenic insult. Thus, its presence is more reminiscent of immune activation than immune suppression.

In summary, we believe that the current concept of a strong local immunosuppression to explain the progression of tumors in the presence of antitumor immunity should be reconsidered in view of recent experimental observations. These observations suggest that antitumor T cell responses continue to be active in the tumor environment, despite their inhibition through several mechanisms, including physiological brakes such as CTLA-4 and PD-1. Owing to the continuous proliferation of tumor cells, the numbers game remains in favor of tumor growth, unless immune intervention tilts the balance.

Conflicts of interest

The authors declare no conflicts of interest.

References

1. Boon, T. & P. van der Bruggen. 1996. Human tumor antigens recognized by T lymphocytes. *J. Exp. Med.* **183:** 725–729.
2. Boon, T., P.G. Coulie, B. Van den Eynde, *et al.* 2006. Human T cell responses against melanoma. *Annu. Rev. Immunol.* **24:** 175–208.
3. Coulie, P.G., V. Karanikas, D. Colau, *et al.* 2001. A monoclonal cytolytic T-lymphocyte response observed in a melanoma patient vaccinated with a tumor-specific antigenic peptide encoded by gene MAGE-3. *Proc. Natl. Acad. Sci. U.S.A.* **98:** 10290–10295.
4. Karanikas, V., C. Lurquin, D. Colau, *et al.* 2003. Monoclonal anti-MAGE-3 CTL responses in melanoma patients displaying tumor regression after vaccination with a recombinant canarypox virus. *J. Immunol.* **171:** 4898–4904.
5. Germeau, C., W. Ma, F. Schiavetti, *et al.* 2005. High frequency of anti-tumor T cells in the blood of melanoma patients before and after vaccination with tumor antigens. *J. Exp. Med.* **201:** 241–248.
6. Gajewski, T.F., Y. Meng, C. Blank, *et al.* 2006. Immune resistance orchestrated by the tumor microenvironment. *Immunol. Rev.* **213:** 131–145.
7. Hodi, F.S., S.J. O'Day, D.F. McDermott, *et al.* 2010. Improved survival with ipilimumab in patients with metastatic melanoma. *N. Engl. J. Med.* **363:** 711–723.
8. Topalian, S.L., F.S. Hodi, J.R. Brahmer, *et al.* 2012. Safety, activity, and immune correlates of anti-PD-1 antibody in cancer. *N. Engl. J. Med.* **366:** 2443–2454.
9. Pages, F., J. Galon, M.C. Dieu-Nosjean, *et al.* 2010. Immune infiltration in human tumors: a prognostic factor that should not be ignored. *Oncogene* **29:** 1093–1102.
10. Cipponi, A., M. Mercier, T. Seremet, *et al.* 2012. Neogenesis of lymphoid structures and antibody responses occur in human melanoma metastases. *Cancer Res.* **72:** 3997–4007.
11. Martinet, L., I. Garrido, T. Filleron, *et al.* 2011. Human solid tumors contain high endothelial venules: association with T- and B-lymphocyte infiltration and favorable prognosis in breast cancer. *Cancer Res.* **71:** 5678–5687.

12. Dieu-Nosjean, M.C., M. Antoine, C. Danel, *et al.* 2008. Long-term survival for patients with non-small-cell lung cancer with intratumoral lymphoid structures. *J. Clin. Oncol.* **26:** 4410–4417.

13. Messina, J.L., D.A. Fenstermacher, S. Eschrich, *et al.* 2012. 12-Chemokine gene signature identifies lymph node-like structures in melanoma: potential for patient selection for immunotherapy? *Sci. Rep.* **2.** Article number 765.

14. Stockis, J., W. Fink, V. Francois, *et al.* 2009. Comparison of stable human Treg and Th clones by transcriptional profiling. *Eur. J. Immunol.* **39:** 869–882.

15. Linterman, M.A., W. Pierson, S.K. Lee, *et al.* 2011. Foxp3$^+$ follicular regulatory T cells control the germinal center response. *Nat. Med.* **17:** 975–982.

16. Chung, Y., S. Tanaka, F. Chu, *et al.* 2011. Follicular regulatory T cells expressing Foxp3 and Bcl-6 suppress germinal center reactions. *Nat. Med.* **17:** 983–988.

Ann. N.Y. Acad. Sci. ISSN 0077-8923

ANNALS OF THE NEW YORK ACADEMY OF SCIENCES

Issue: *The Renaissance of Cancer Immunotherapy*

Main features of human T helper 17 cells

Francesco Annunziato, Lorenzo Cosmi, Francesco Liotta, Enrico Maggi, and Sergio Romagnani

Laboratory of Immunology, Allergology and Cellular Therapies, Department of Internal Medicine and Denothe Center, University of Florence, Italy

Address for correspondence: Sergio Romagnani, Laboratory of Immunology, Allergology and Cellular Therapies, Department of Internal Medicine, University of Florence, Complesso Polivalente, Viale Pieraccini 6, Firenze 50139-Italy. s.romagnani@dmi.unifi.it

In addition to T helper type 1 (Th1) and Th2 cells, Th17 cells are a third arm of effector $CD4^+$ T cells. Human Th17 cells express RORC and CD161 and originate from RORC-expressing $CD161^+$ precursors, which migrate to lymphoid tissue and differentiate into mature Th17 cells in response to interleukin (IL)-1β and IL-23. Human Th17 cells are rare in inflamed tissues for two reasons: (1) Th17 cells do not produce IL-2 and, therefore, do not proliferate in response to TCR signaling, mainly because of RORC-dependent IL-4I1–mediated mechanisms that interfere with IL-2 gene activation; and (2) Th17 cell shift to a Th1 phenotype in the presence of IL-12; such Th17-derived Th1 cells are considered to be nonclassical Th1 cells and can be distinguished from classical Th1 cells. The possible role of Th17 cells in human tumors is still unclear and even controversial.

Keywords: Th17; CXCL8; RORC; IL-4I1; nonclassic Th1

Introduction

Effector $CD4^+$ T helper (Th) cells have been distinguished into different lineages based on their pattern of cytokine secretion, transcription factor expression, and functions, which are responsible for both different types of protection, as well as of immunopathology. Th1 cells produce interferon (IFN)-γ, express the transcription factor T-bet, protect against intracellular infections, and have been implicated in the pathogenesis of organ-specific autoimmune disorders. Th2 cells produce interleukin (IL)-4, IL-5, and IL-13, express the transcription factor GATA-3, protect against helminthes, and are involved in the pathogenesis of allergic (atopic) disorders.[1,2] A third subset of $CD4^+$ effector T cells, Th17 cells, has been characterized in recent years; these $CD4^+$ T cells produce IL-17 and other cytokines when they are stimulated. Murine Th17 cells express the transcription factor RORγt, protect against infections sustained by extracellular bacteria and fungi, and, because of their ability to activate macrophages and also to recruit neutrophil granulocytes, have been suspected to play an important role in the pathogenesis of different chronic inflammatory disorders.[3,4] Although there are many similarities between murine and human Th17 cells, there are also some phenotypic and functional differences.

Activities of human Th17 cells

Like murine Th17 cells, human Th17 cells produce IL-17A and IL-17F, and these cytokines have been used to define this subset. Human Th17 cells also produce other cytokines, such as IL-21, IL-22, and IL-26, but also tumor necrosis factor (TNF)-α and granulocyte-monocyte colony stimulatory factor (GM-CSF). IL-17A induces the production of the chemokine CXC ligand (CXCL)8 from epithelial cells, endothelial cells, fibroblasts, and macrophages, leading to the recruitment of neutrophil granulocytes.[5] Human Th17 cells themselves have been found to be able to directly produce CXCL8.[6] In murine models, production of IFN-γ and IL-4 by Th1 and Th2 cells, respectively, was found to be antagonistic to the production of IL-17A.[6]

In previously published work we showed in $CD4^+$ T cells infiltrating the mucosa of patients with Crohn's diseases the presence of high numbers of

doi: 10.1111/nyas.12075

 Ann. N.Y. Acad. Sci. 1284 (2013) 66–70 © 2013 New York Academy of Sciences.

CD4[+] T cells producing both IL-17A and IFN-γ, which we referred to as "Th17–Th1" cells. In addition, Th17 clones that produced IL-17A but not IFN-γ *in vitro* could be shifted to produce of IFN-γ in cultures containing IL-12.[7] In a subsequent study we demonstrated the existence of small proportions of CD4[+] T cells able to produce both IL-17A and IL-4 (Th17–Th2 cells), which were more abundant in the peripheral blood of patients with severe chronic asthma; and Th17–Th2 cells could be generated *in vitro* by culturing Th17 clones in the presence of IL-4.[8] These findings suggest that under certain conditions Th17 cells exhibit plasticity and shift to the production of type 1 or type 2 cytokines (see below).

Origin of human Th17 cells

Although murine Th17 cells originate from naive T helper cells in response to the combined activity of IL-6 and transforming growth factor (TGF)-β,[9] the latter cytokine has not been found to be essential for the differentiation of human Th17 cells.[10–12] Although this discrepancy was initially attributed to the unrecognized presence of TGF-β in serum-containing cultures,[13] subsequent studies showed that human Th17 differentiation could also be obtained in serum-free medium that included IL-1β and IL-23. More importantly, after it was found that all memory human Th17 cells express the natural killer (NK) and NKT marker CD161,[14] the existence of Th17 precursors were identified in both the umbilical cord blood (UCB) and newborn thymus. These CD161[+] T cell precursors, which were not present in the adult peripheral blood, expressed RORC, IL-23 receptor, and CCR6, and were able to differentiate into mature IL-17A–producing cells only when cultured in the combined presence of IL-1β and IL-23, even in the absence of TGF-β.[14] Subsequently, our group found that CD161 is expressed not only by CD4[+] T cells, but also by CD8[+] and double-negative (CD4[−]CD8[−]) T cells, able to produce IL-17A, and in their UCB precursors.[15] These findings suggest that human Th17 cells originate from a distinct lineage of CD161[+] RORC-expressing T cell precursors already present in the human thymus, which then directly migrate to lymphoid tissues where they can develop into mature Th17 cells under the combined activity of IL-1β and IL-23.[5] More recent studies performed in mice have also shown the dispens-

ability of TGF-β, as well as the essential role of IL-1β and IL-23, in the orchestration of Th17 cell differentiation.[16–19]

Reasons for rarity of human Th17 cells in the inflammatory sites

Despite the importance of their pathogenic role in different human pathological conditions, Th17 cells are very difficult to detect in the inflamed tissues. The rarity of human Th17 cells in inflammatory sites may be explained by their limited expansion in response to T cell receptor (TCR) triggering and their ability to shift to a Th1 phenotype in the presence of IL-12.

Human Th17 cells do not expand in response to TCR triggering

In a recent study, we demonstrated that human Th17 cells proliferate in response to stimulation with PMA plus ionomycin, but not in response to stimulation with anti-CD3 plus anti-CD28 monoclonal antibodies (anti-CD3/CD28 mAb).[20] This difference was mainly due to the lack of IL-2 production by Th17 cells and to their reduced capacity to respond to this cytokine; for example, the addition of exogenous IL-2 to cultures of Th17 cells stimulated with anti-CD3/CD28 mAb only partially restored their proliferation.[20] In searching

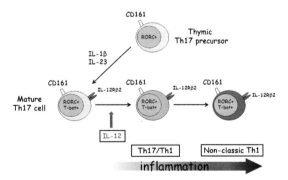

Figure 1. Origin and destiny of human Th17 cells. Precursors of Th17 cells are contained within a small subset of thymic CD161[+] cells, which also express RORC, but not IL-17A mRNA. These cells enter the circulation during both ontogeny and the early stages of childhood and directly migrate to mucosal lymphoid tissues. Here, under inflammatory conditions that are characterized by the production of IL-1β and IL-23, they acquire the ability to produce IL-17A, thus becoming mature Th17 cells. Then, in the presence of IL-12, Th17 cells acquire the ability to produce IFN-γ in addition to IL-17A (Th17/Th1) and then become "nonclassical" Th1 cells.

for the mechanism responsible for the inability of human Th17 cells to produce IL-2 in response to TCR triggering, we found a significant reduction in the phosphorylation of the IL-2 promoter–binding transcription factors c-Jun and c-Fos, as well as reduced NFAT nuclear translocation and lower NFAT activity, in Th17 cells compared with Th1 cells, whereas no differences in the phosphorylation of NF-κB were observed.[20] The expression of CD3ζ and ε chains, as well as phosphorylation of CD3ζ, ZAP70 and SLP76, were also found to be significantly lower in Th17 cells compared with Th1 cells.[20] We also found that Th17 cells exhibit strong up-regulation of the IL-4–induced gene 1 (*IL4I1*), which is virtually inactivated in Th1 cells.[20] IL4I1, a phenylalanine oxidase known to be produced by B lymphocytes[21] and dendritic cells (DC),[22] is able to inhibit T cell proliferation via the enzymatic production of H_2O_2, which results in decreased CD3ζ chain expression.[22] Interestingly, *IL4I1* was found to be up-regulated not only in memory Th17 cells but also in their UCB and thymic precursors.[20] The direct demonstration of the role of the *IL4I1* up-regulation in the inability of human Th17 cells to produce IL-2 and to proliferate in response to TCR triggering was provided by the observation that RORC silencing reduced *IL4I1* expression and enabled Th17 cells to proliferate in response to TCR triggering. Moreover, RT-PCR on DNA from Th17 cell clones precipitated with a RORC Ab, performed with *IL4I1*-specific promoter primers indicated the direct interaction between RORC and *IL4I1*.[20] Thus, a RORC-dependent upregulation of *IL4I1* is mainly responsible for the limited expansion of human Th17 cells in response to TCR triggering.

Human Th17 cells rapidly shift to the Th1 phenotype in presence of IL-12

The limited ability of human Th17 cells to proliferate in response to TCR triggering is perhaps not the only reason for the rarity of human Th17 cells in inflammatory sites. The possibility of plasticity of human Th17 cells—to become more Th1- or Th2-like—may also contribute to their being found infrequently in inflammatory sites.

As mentioned previously, we showed *in vitro* that Th17 clones can begin producing IFN-γ in addition to IL-17A;[7] and in a subsequent study performed on the synovial fluid (SF) of patients affected by juvenile idiopathic arthritis (JIA), we found an accumulation of CD161⁺CD4⁺ T cells among which were very few Th17 cells, whereas the majority of the CD161⁺CD4⁺ T cells produced both IL-17A and IFN-γ, or IFN-γ alone.[23] When purified Th17 cells from the SF of these patients were cultured *in vitro* in medium alone, they spontaneously shifted to a Th1 phenotype; also, purified Th17 cells from peripheral blood of healthy subjects, which maintain their cytokine profile when cultured in medium alone, rapidly shifted to a Th1 phenotype if cultured in the presence of IL-12 or the SF of JIA patients. Of note was a direct correlation between the numbers of CD161⁺CD4⁺ T cells present in the SF of JIA patients and two parameters of disease activity, such as the erythrocyte sedimentation rate and the level of C-reactive protein.[23] Thus, it seems that at least in JIA, Th17-derived Th1 cells play an important

Table 1. Main features of human Th17, classic, and nonclassic Th1 cells

	Th17	Classic Th1	Nonclassic Th1
Origin	CD161⁺ RORC⁺ thymic precursors	CD161⁻ naive Th	CD161⁺ RORC⁺ thymic precursors Th17 cells
Polarizing cytokines	IL-1β + IL-23	IL-12	IL-1β + IL-23; IL-12
Site of maturation	Mucosal lymphoid tissues	Lymph nodes	Inflammatory sites
Transcription factors	RORC^high T-bet^low	T-bet	T-bet^high RORC^low
Chemokine receptors	CCR6, CCR4	CXCR3	CXCR3, CCR6
Cytokine receptor	IL-1β, -23, -12, -17C	IL-12	IL-1β, -23, -12, -17C
CD28	+++	+	+++
CD161	+++	−	+++
IL4I1	+++	−	+++

role in the inflammatory process; these Th1 cells are referred to as nonclassical to distinguish them from the classical Th1 cells (Fig. 1). In a subsequent study, some features of classical and nonclassical Th1 cells were examined; nonclassical Th1 cells can be distinguished from classical Th1 cells because of the expression by nonclassical Th1 cells of CD161, RORC, CCR6, IL-17RE, and IL4I1 (Table 1).[24]

Role of Th17 cells in human tumors and in antitumor vaccination

The role of Th17 cells has been investigated, but the results obtained so far are still unclear and even controversial. An imbalance between Th17 cells and T regulatory (T$_{reg}$) cells seems to be associated with poor prognosis in melanoma and in prostatic and ovarian cancers,[25–27] and low levels of IL-17 have been reported to indicate poor prognosis in gastric adenocarcinoma;[28] such findings suggest a possible protective role of Th17 cells against cancer. This possibility has been supported by experiments performed in mice with ovarian cancer, where it was shown that immunization with attenuated activated syngeneic T cells led to augmentation of antitumor immunity accompanied by dampened T$_{reg}$ cell function and increased Th17 cell development.[29] However, prevalence of the Th17 phenotype was found in gastric cancer tissue, suggesting that these cells may rather play a role in the gastric cancer progression.[30] One major problem is the respective role of Th17 cells, as well as of classic and nonclassic Th1 cells, in either protection or progression, which still needs to be solved.

Conflict of interest

The authors declare no conflicts of interest.

References

1. Mosmann, T.R. & R.L. Coffman. 1989. TH1 And TH2 cells: different patterns of lymphokine secretion lead to different functional properties. *Annu. Rev. Immunol.* **7:** 145–173
2. Romagnani, S. 1994. Lymphokine production by human T cells in disease states. *Annu. Rev. Immunol.* **12:** 227–257.
3. Cosmi, L., F. Liotta, E. Maggi, *et al.* 2011. Th17 cells: new players in asthma pathogenesis. *Allergy* **66:** 989–998.
4. Annunziato, F., L. Cosmi, F. Liotta, *et al.* 2008. The phenotype of human Th17 cells and their precursors, the cytokines that mediate their differentiation and the role of Th17 cells in inflammation. *Int. Immunol.* **20:** 1361–1368.
5. Annunziato, F., L. Cosmi, F. Liotta, *et al.* 2012. Defining the human T helper 17 cell phenotype. *Trends Immunol.* **33:** 505–512.

6. Pelletier, M., L. Maggi, A. Micheletti, *et al.* 2010. Evidence for a cross-talk between human neutrophils and Th17 cells. *Blood* **115:** 335–343.
7. Annunziato, F., L. Cosmi, V. Santarlasci, *et al.* 2007. Phenotypic and functional features of human Th17 cells. *J. Exp. Med.* **204:** 1849–1861.
8. Cosmi, L., L. Maggi, V. Santarlasci, *et al.* 2010. Identification of a novel subset of human circulating memory CD4(+. T cells that produce both IL-17A and IL-4. *J. Allergy Clin. Immunol.* **125:** 222–230.
9. Bettelli, E., Y. Carrier, W. Gao, *et al.* 2006. Reciprocal developmental pathways for the generation of pathogenic effector TH17 and regulatory T cells. *Nature* **441:** 235–238.
10. Acosta Rodriguez, E.V., G. Napolitani, A. Lanzavecchia & F. Sallusto. 2007. Surface phenotype and antigen specificity of human interleukin 17-producing T helper memory cells. *Nat. Immunol.* **8:** 639–646.
11. Wilson, N.J., K. Boniface, J.R. Chan, *et al.* 2007. Development, cytokine profile and function of human interleukin 17-producing helper T cells. *Nat. Immunol.* **8:** 950–957.
12. Chen, Z., C.M. Tato, L. Muul, *et al.* 2007. Distinct regulation of interleukin-17 in human T helper lymphocytes. *Arthritis Rheum.* **56:** 2936–2946.
13. Santarlasci, V., L. Maggi, M. Capone, *et al.* 2009). TGF-beta indirectly favors the development of human Th17 cells by inhibiting Th1 cells. *Eur. J. Immunol.* **39:** 207–215.
14. Cosmi, L., R. De Palma, V. Santarlasci, *et al.* 2008. Human interleukin 17-producing cells originate from a CD161$^+$CD4$^+$ T cell precursor. *J. Exp. Med.* **205:** 1903–1916.
15. Maggi, L., V. Santarlasci, M. Capone, *et al.* 2010. CD161 is a marker of all human IL-17-producing T-cell subsets and is induced by RORC. *Eur. J. Immunol.* **40:** 2174–2181.
16. Chung, Y., S.H. Chang, G.J. Martinez, *et al.* 2009. Critical regulation of early Th17 cell differentiation by interleukin-1 signaling. *Immunity* **30:** 576–587.
17. Ghoreschi, K., A. Laurence, X.P. Yang, *et al.* 2010. Generation of pathogenic T(H)17 cells in the absence of TGF-beta signalling. *Nature* **467:** 967–971.
18. Marks, B.R., H.N. Nowyhed, J.Y. Choi, *et al.* 2009. Thymic self-reactivity selects natural interleukin 17-producing T cells that can regulate peripheral inflammation. *Nat. Immunol.* **10:** 1125–1132.
19. Kim, J.S., J.E. Smith-Garvin, G.A. Koretzky & M.S. Jordan. 2011. The requirements for natural Th17 cell development are distinct from those of conventional Th17 cells. *J. Exp. Med.* **208:** 2201–2207.
20. Santarlasci, V., L. Maggi, M. Capone, *et al.* 2012. Rarity of human T helper 17 cells is due to retinoic acid orphan receptor-dependent mechanisms that limit their expansion. *Immunity* **36:** 201–214.
21. Chu, C.C. & W.E. Paul. 1998. Expressed genes in interleukin-4 treated B cells identified by cDNA representational difference analysis. *Mol. Immunol.* **35:** 487–502.
22. Boulland, M.L., J. Marquet, V. Molinier-Frenkel, *et al.* 2007. Human IL4I1 is a secreted L-phenylalanine oxidase expressed by mature dendritic cells that inhibits T-lymphocyte proliferation. *Blood* **110:** 220–227.

23. Cosmi, L., R. Cimaz, L. Maggi, *et al.* 2011. Evidence of the transient nature of the Th17 phenotype of CD4$^+$CD161$^+$ T cells in the synovial fluid of patients with juvenile idiopathic arthritis. *Arthritis Rheum.* **63:** 2504–2515.

24. Maggi, L., V. Santarlasci, M. Capone, *et al.* 2012. Distinctive features of classic and non-classic (Th17-derived) human Th1 cells. *Eur. J. Immunol.* **42:** 3180–3188.

25. Kryczek, I., S. Wei, L. Zou, *et al.* 2007. Cutting edge: Th17 and regulatory T cell dynamics and the regulation by IL-2 in the tumor microenvironment. *J. Immunol.* **178:** 6730–6733.

26. Sfanos, K.S., T.C. Bruno, C.H. Maris, *et al.* 2008. Phenotypic analysis of prostate-infiltrating lymphocytes reveals TH17 and Treg skewing. *Clin. Cancer Res.* **14:** 3254–3261.

27. Kryczek, I., M. Banerjee, P. Cheng, *et al.* 2009. Phenotype, distribution, generation, and functional and clinical relevance of Th17 cells in the human tumor environments. *Blood* **114:** 1141–1149.

28. Chen, J.G., J.C. Xia, X.T. Liang, *et al.* 2011. Intratumoral expression of IL-17 and its prognostic role in gastric adenocarcinoma patients. *Int. J. Biol. Sci.* **7:** 53–60.

29. Wang, L., J. Lin, Z. Zhou, *et al.* 2011. Up-regulation of Th17 cells may underlined inhibition of Treg development caused by immunization with activated syngeneic T cells. *Plos One* **6:** 1–12.

30. Yamada, Y., H. Saito & M. Ikeguchi. 2012. Prevalence and clinical relevance of Th17 cells in patients with gastric cancer. *J. Surg. Res.* **178:** 685–691.

Ann. N.Y. Acad. Sci. ISSN 0077-8923

ANNALS OF THE NEW YORK ACADEMY OF SCIENCES

Issue: *The Renaissance of Cancer Immunotherapy*

In silico modeling of cancer cell dissemination and metastasis

Lu-En Wai, Vipin Narang, Alexandre Gouaillard, Lai Guan Ng, and Jean-Pierre Abastado

Singapore Immunology Network (SIgN), Agency for Science, Technology and Research (A*STAR), Biopolis, Singapore

Address for correspondence: Jean-Pierre Abastado, Lab of Tumour Immunology, Singapore Immunology Network (SIgN), 8A Biomedical Grove, #04-06 Immunos, Singapore 138648. abastado@immunol.a-star.edu.sg

Metastasis is the main cause of cancer-related death. It is surprising then that the exact nature of metastasis—the process by which cancer cells leave the primary tumor to reach distant organs, and resume proliferation—is not fully understood. Moreover, the different conditions under which the immune system can either promote or suppress metastasis are only now beginning to be uncovered. In recent years, our understanding of metastasis as a genocentric, cell-autonomous process has shifted toward a systemic model in which interactions between cancer cells and their surrounding microenvironments lead to dissemination and metastasis. *In silico* modeling of the various steps involved in metastasis can help provide an understanding of how tumor properties emerge from the complex interplays between tumor cells and their microenvironment. *In silico* models can also be useful in identifying the selective forces that favor the outcomes of cancer cells with metastatic potential.

Keywords: modeling; cancer; metastasis; epithelial–mesenchymal transition

Cancer cells disseminate early

Cancer is the second leading cause of global human mortality. Early cancers can be cured relatively efficiently, but once metastases develop in distant organs, most cancers become fatal. Surprisingly, recent studies in mice and humans have shown that cancer cell dissemination is an early event that usually takes place before the primary tumor can be detected clinically.[1,2] By extension, the majority of human cancer patients have cancer cells already disseminated throughout their body when their cancer gets diagnosed, yet a large proportion of these patients can still be successfully cured. It is not clear why disseminated cancer cells only rarely develop into overt metastases in this patient group. However, it is apparent that the immune system plays an important role in restricting metastasis development, since dormant cancer cells can resume proliferation when the host is immunosuppressed, as in cases of organ transplantation.[3–5]

The role of the tumor stroma

Thirty years ago, the discovery of oncogenes and tumor suppressor genes led to the genocentric view that cancer is a cell-autonomous disease caused by accumulation of genetic and epigenetic alterations in cancer cells.[6] This view has prevailed for several decades, but largely ignores previous observations showing that the tumor microenvironment can control cancer cells. For example, aggregation of teratocarcinoma cells with blastocyst leads to dominant suppression of their oncogenic potential, and normal chimeric mice can be obtained following injection of embryonal carcinoma cells into blastocysts.[7] More recently, H.L. Moses and colleagues showed that loss of TGF-β responsiveness in fibroblasts by conditional inactivation of TGF-β–receptor 2 results in intraepithelial neoplasia of the prostate and invasive squamous cell carcinoma of the fore-stomach.[8] Similarly, specific gene deletion of *Dicer1* or *Sbds* in mesenchymal stromal cells alters hematopoiesis and results in myeloproliferative disorders, leading to secondary acute myeloid leukemia (AML) in some mice.[9] The role of the tumor stroma in the development and progression of cancer is now widely appreciated and novel therapeutic strategies that target the tumor stroma are currently in development.[10]

doi: 10.1111/nyas.12077

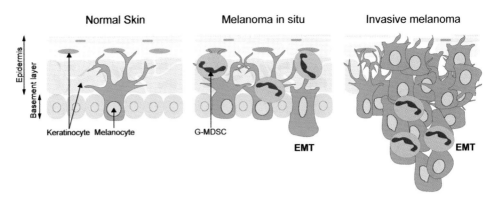

Figure 1. Early dissemination of cancer cells. Granulocytic myeloid-derived suppressor cells (G-MDSC) infiltrate the primary tumor and induce epithelial–mesenchymal transition (EMT) in the early stages of melanoma development. Cancer cells that have undergone EMT grow faster and disseminate to distant sites. Data are adapted from Refs. 13 and 14.

The role of immune microenvironment

Immune cells in the tumor microenvironment play a significant role in modulating tumor growth and cancer progression. Tumor-associated macrophages produce trophic factors and are essential for the growth of new blood vessels.[11] Macrophages are also directly involved in cancer cell motility, especially in intra- and extravasation.[12] We have shown that a subset of myeloid cells, the granulocytic myeloid-derived suppressor cells (G-MDSC), promotes cancer cell proliferation and dissemination.[13] In a mouse model of spontaneous melanoma (the RE-TAAD transgenic mouse), G-MDSCs preferentially accumulate in the primary tumor where they induce epithelial–mesenchymal transition (EMT)—an integrated program in which epithelial cells reduce their contacts with neighboring cells, change shape, and acquire a motile phenotype (Fig. 1). The EMT process has been extensively described during embryogenesis as well as in *in vitro* systems. We showed that, in cocultures with G-MDSC, various cancer cells undergo EMT and become highly motile. We have also provided evidence that EMT occurs in tumors *in vivo*, and demonstrated that G-MDSC depletion can reduce EMT, impair cancer cell dissemination, and restrict metastasis.

Selection of metastatic cells

If disseminated cancer cells can remain dormant for months or even years, what are the selective pressures that eventually initiate EMT and promote metastasis? To address this question, we developed an *in silico* agent-based model that simulates tumor growth.[14] In this model, each cell was ascribed defined probabilities of undergoing cell death or cell division, depending on nutrient availability. Other cell properties, including rate of nutrient consumption, cell motility, and adhesion to neighboring cells or to the extracellular matrix, were also defined. By varying these parameters, virtual cells could be classified as either epithelial-like (high adhesion, low motility) or mesenchymal-like (low adhesion, high motility) and were able to switch from epithelial to mesenchymal phenotype (EMT). We found that where access to nutrients was limited, mesenchymal-like cells had a growth advantage over epithelial-like cells. Tumors made of mesenchymal cells grew faster and larger than those composed of epithelial cells. Moreover, when only one cell in a growing epithelial tumor was allowed to undergo EMT and adopt a mesenchymal phenotype, the mesenchymal progeny typically overgrew the epithelial cells and the whole tumor became mesenchymal. Our *in silico* model suggests that highly motile cells have a growth advantage within the primary tumor, and that progressive selection of these motile populations increases the overall likelihood of metastasis. Importantly, this advantage was only observed if nutrients were limiting.

Our *in silico* model may explain the relative failure of therapeutic strategies that aim to starve tumors of nutrients. Despite the initial excitement surrounding the therapeutic potential of anti-angiogenic drugs, the performance of these treatments in clinical testing has been disappointing. Although anti-angiogenic therapy can induce tumor regression in isolated cases, such approaches have been shown to

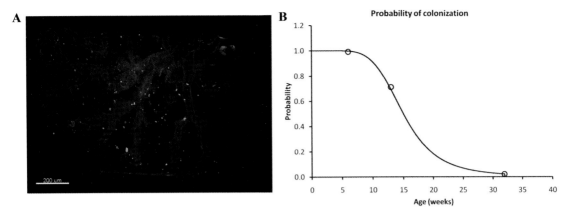

Figure 2. The probability of successful colonization of the lung decreases with age. (A) The number and size distribution of lung micrometastases are determined experimentally at various ages using ultramicroscopy. A representative lung lobe is shown, with tumor cells in green and lung morphology in red. (B) The probability of successful colonization is determined by fitting experimental data with an *in silico* model. The probabilities determined at three time points are depicted as circles on the graph. Data are from Wai *et al.* (in preparation).

eventually select for aggressive tumor variants with higher risk of metastasis.[15]

Our *in silico* model yielded a further unexpected result: tumors comprised of mesenchymal cells exhibit a multinodular structure, whereas tumors made of epithelial cells are more compact. Macroscopic tumor morphology thus appears to be an emergent characteristic of tumors that is determined by the individual properties of the constituent cells. Using RETAAD mice, we were able to verify experimentally that depletion of G-MDSC reduced tumor nodularity. The association of mesenchymal transition with increased tumor nodularity may explain why multinodular tumors are associated with a poorer prognosis in certain cancers.[16]

Patterns of tumor dissemination and niche colonization

Cancer cell dissemination is only the first step of the metastatic process. To develop into macroscopic tumors, disseminated cancer cells need to reach the target organ, survive in this ectopic location, and resume proliferation. As the primary tumor grows, it secretes factors that modify the distant organ in such a way that it becomes more hospitable to disseminated cancer cells. These modifications of the target organ create sites where disseminated cancer cells can survive and eventually resume proliferation more efficiently. Such sites are referred to as metastatic niches.

To dissect this process and explore the possible roles of immune cells, we have developed a second *in silico* statistical model that recapitulates the various steps of metastasis. In agreement with measurements of circulating cancer cells in cancer patients, we postulate that dissemination mirrors the primary tumor growth. We also assume that tumor growth at the ectopic location followed a Gompertzian curve. Using ultramicroscopy to image entire lungs, we have determined the number and size of lung metastases in RETAAD mice at different ages and then compared predictions of the *in silico* model with the experimental measurements (Fig. 2A, Wai *et al.*, in preparation). We found that the probability of cancer cell seeding and successful colonization of the lung decreased with time (Fig. 2B, Wai *et al.*, in preparation). This decrease could be explained in two ways. First, the intrinsic ability of cancer cells to initiate metastasis could decrease with age, resulting in fewer metastasis-initiating cells being released into the circulation even as the primary tumor grows. Second, the probability of disseminated cancer cells finding a niche could decrease with age. Given a finite number of niches, additional cancer cells would be less likely to successfully occupy a target organ as niches fill up. Regardless of explanation, our finding that successful colonization of the lung decreases with time and has an important consequence on our understanding of metastasis development. We already knew that cancer cell dissemination occurs early during cancer development.

This new finding indicates that metastases develop mostly from these early disseminating cancer cells.

Conclusion

Metastasis is not merely a consequence of the accumulation of random mutations that instill cancer cells with the ability to colonize remote anatomical sites. Cancer cell dissemination is an early event, and disseminated cancer cells can remain dormant for prolonged periods of time. Myeloid immune cells that infiltrate the primary tumor modulate the properties of the constituent cancer cells. Data from our *in silico* model suggest that metastatic cancer cells have a growth advantage when nutrient supplies are limited, as is the case in small tumors that have yet to undergo angiogenic switch. Dissemination of cancer cells to distant organs can thus be considered a byproduct of the selective advantage conferred by high cell motility.

Once cancer cells reach the target organ, they survive and resume proliferation only if they encounter a proper microenvironment, referred to as a niche. We showed that the development of these niches is temporally regulated. In our mouse model, the number of niches seems to decrease sharply with age. Immune cells are also likely to play a role in niche formation. Our long-term goal is to identify cellular or molecular players that determine the fate of disseminated cancer cells.

The conclusions drawn from our models must be issued with a note of caution—these models are simplified representations of the complex process that takes place during tumor growth and morphogenesis. A limited number of hypotheses were incorporated into our models so that computational requirements remained manageable, hence further experimental data will now be required to evaluate our findings. However, we do believe that our models provide a conceptual framework that can account for several phenomena observed in real biological systems. We hope that our findings will help guide oncologists toward a better understanding of the mechanisms that drive the lethal process of metastasis.

Acknowledgments

This research was funded by SIgN, A*STAR, Singapore. The authors wish to thank Neil McCarthy of Insight Editing London for manuscript editing.

Conflicts of interest

The authors declare no conflicts of interest.

References

1. Eyles, J. *et al.* 2010. Tumor cells disseminate early, but immunosurveillance limits metastatic outgrowth, in a mouse model of melanoma. *J. Clin. Invest.* **120:** 2030–2039.
2. Rhim, A.D. *et al.* 2012. EMT and dissemination precede pancreatic tumor formation. *Cell* **148:** 349–361.
3. Milton, C.A. *et al.* 2006. The transmission of donor-derived malignant melanoma to a renal allograft recipient. *Clin. Transplant.* **20:** 547–550.
4. Koebel, C.M. *et al.* 2007. Adaptive immunity maintains occult cancer in an equilibrium state. *Nature* **450:** 903–907.
5. Lu, X. *et al.* 2011. VCAM-1 promotes osteolytic expansion of indolent bone micrometastasis of breast cancer by engaging alpha4beta1-positive osteoclast progenitors. *Cancer Cell* **20:** 701–714.
6. Hanahan, D. & R.A. Weinberg. 2000. The hallmarks of cancer. *Cell* **100:** 57–70.
7. Papaioannou, V.E. *et al.* 1975. Fate of teratocarcinoma cells injected into early mouse embryos. *Nature* **258:** 70–73.
8. Bhowmick, N.A. *et al.* 2004. TGF-beta signaling in fibroblasts modulates the oncogenic potential of adjacent epithelia. *Science* **303:** 848–851.
9. Raaijmakers, M.H. *et al.* 2010. Bone progenitor dysfunction induces myelodysplasia and secondary leukaemia. *Nature* **464:** 852–857.
10. Engels, B., D.A. Rowley & H. Schreiber. 2012. Targeting stroma to treat cancers. *Semin. Cancer Biol.* **22:** 41–49.
11. Qian, B.Z. & J.W. Pollard. 2010. Macrophage diversity enhances tumor progression and metastasis. *Cell* **141:** 39–51.
12. Wyckoff, J.B. *et al.* 2007. Direct visualization of macrophage-assisted tumor cell intravasation in mammary tumors. *Cancer Res.* **67:** 2649–2656.
13. Toh, B. *et al.* 2011. Mesenchymal transition and dissemination of cancer cells is driven by myeloid-derived suppressor cells infiltrating the primary tumor. *PLoS Biol.* **9:** e1001162.
14. Narang, V. *et al.* 2012. Selection of mesenchymal-like metastatic cells in primary tumors—an in silico investigation. *Front Immunol.* **3:** 88.
15. Paez-Ribes, M. *et al.* 2009. Antiangiogenic therapy elicits malignant progression of tumors to increased local invasion and distant metastasis. *Cancer Cell* **15:** 220–231.
16. Pons, F., M. Varela & J.M. Llovet. 2005. Staging systems in hepatocellular carcinoma. *HPB (Oxford)* **7:** 35–41.

Ann. N.Y. Acad. Sci. ISSN 0077-8923

ANNALS OF THE NEW YORK ACADEMY OF SCIENCES
Issue: *The Renaissance of Cancer Immunotherapy*

Common pathways to tumor rejection

Ena Wang,[1] Davide Bedognetti,[1,2,3] Sara Tomei,[1,4] and Francesco M. Marincola[1,4]

[1]Infectious Disease and Immunogenetics Section (IDIS), Department of Transfusion Medicine, Clinical Center and trans-NIH Center for Human Immunology (CHI), National Institutes of Health, Bethesda, Maryland. [2]Department of Oncology, Biology Genetics (DOBIG), University of Genoa and National Cancer Research Institute, Genoa, Italy. [3]Department of Internal Medicine (DiMI), University of Genoa, Genoa, Italy. [4]Chief Research Office, Sidra Medical and Research Center, Doha, Qatar

Address for correspondence: Francesco M. Marincola, Chief Research Officer, Sidra Medical and Research Center, P.O. Box 26999, Doha, Qatar. fmarincola@mail.cc.nih.gov

The control of tumor growth by the host's immunosurveillance is centered on the activation of interferon (IFN) pathways. In particular, direct study of tumors by various groups has uncovered an IFN-γ–related signature whose presence is consistently associated with better prognosis, predisposition to respond to immunotherapy, and, in its extreme manifestation, the acute phases of tumor rejection. Together, and related to the IFN-γ–associated signature, a cluster of genes are coordinately expressed that we refer to as the *immunologic constant of rejection* (ICR). Activation of ICR components is observed in all forms of immune-mediated, tissue-specific destruction, including autoimmunity, allograft rejection, graft-versus-host disease, and killing of affected cells during the acute phases of infection that leads to clearance of pathogens. Thus, tumor rejection is a facet of a general and conserved mechanism that favors (tumor rejection, clearance of pathogen) or encumbers (graft rejection, autoimmunity) the organism. Here, we summarize progress in the understanding of its genesis, outline the difficulties, and propose a strategy for understanding the causes of tumor rejection.

Keywords: cancer immunotherapy; melanoma; rejection; autoimmunity

Introduction

It is a recurrent theme that the control of tumor growth by the host's immunosurveillance is centered on the activation of interferon (IFN) pathways. In particular, direct study of tumors by various groups has uncovered an IFN-γ–related signature whose presence is consistently associated with various facets of immunosurveillance, such as better prognosis, predisposition to respond to immunotherapy, and the acute phases of tumor rejection. Related to the IFN-γ–associated signature, a cluster of genes are coordinately expressed in all forms of immune-mediated tissue-specific destruction (TSD), including flares of autoimmunity, allograft rejection, graft-versus-host disease, and killing of affected cells during the acute phases of infection that leads to clearance of pathogen; we refer to this coordinate expression as the immunologial constant of rejection (ICR). Tumor rejection is one facet of a general and conserved mechanism that, according to circumstances, favors tumor rejection or clearance of pathogen, or leads to graft rejection or autoimmunity.

Tumor rejection is an aspect of autoimmunity

It has been shown in experimental systems that the host can mount a concerted resistance to tumor growth through the activation of adaptive and innate immune mechanisms.[1] This phenomenon is generally referred to as *immunosurveillance*.[2,3] Among its determinants, the activation of IFN-γ–related genes plays a dominant role.[1] Observational studies performed in humans confirm the relevance of this concept as a biomarker of prognostic[4] and predictive[5–7] value. Biologically related to IFN-γ pathway activation is the coordinate expression of a cluster of genes including interferon-stimulated transcripts such as interferon regulatory factor (IRF)-1; antigen processing and presentation-related genes; several immune effector molecules such as TIA-1, granulysin, granzymes and perforin;

doi: 10.1111/nyas.12063

and; CXCR3 and CCR5 ligand chemokines. We refer to this group of genes as the ICR because expression is consistently observed when a switch from chronic to acute inflammation occurs:[8] to varying degrees of intensity, activation occurs during the acute inflammatory phases associated with all facets of immune-mediated TSD that lead not only to tumor destruction but also to flares of autoimmunity, allograft rejection,[9] graft-versus-host disease,[10] and killing of affected cells during the acute phases of infection, leading to clearance of pathogen. Thus, it seems that a continuous spectrum exists, spanning immunosurveillance that limits the growth of early neoplasms,[11] a limiting effect on the growth of established cancers that affects their prognosis,[4] an immune-activated phenotype likely to respond to immunotherapy,[12, 13] and a full-blown activation of immune effector mechanisms that leads to complete tumor rejection as a tissue-specific form of irrepressible autoimmunity.

Three categories of factors that determine the onset of TSD

Although the biological mechanisms associated with TSD are becoming increasingly accepted, the identity of the determinants that trigger such phenomena in a given individual at a particular time are still unclear. To systematically approach this complex question, it is useful to consider two broad categories of variables that affect the occurrence of TSD: genetic background of the host and exogenous environmental factors. In the case of TSD associated with cancer rejection, a third category should be included, which consists of a set of cancer cell–specific variables, including somatic alterations related to the neoplastic process superimposed on the genetic background of the host and inherited in some proportion by the neoplastic cells, and epigenetic adaptations resulting from tissue-specific ontogeny. The weight played by the genetic background of the host as a determinant/modifier associated with TSD is clearly demonstrated by extensive studies on autoimmune diseases, such as systemic lupus erythematosus.[14] Although less extensively studied, there is emerging evidence that the genetic background of the host is also associated with likelihood of tumor rejection, as recently exemplified by a study from our group in which a polymorphism of IRF-5, well-described to protect from the emergence of systemic lupus erythematosus, was found to be significantly associated with lack of responsiveness of patients with metastatic melanoma to treatment with adoptively transferred tumor-infiltrating lymphocytes.[15] This observation aligns with the well-established association of emergence of autoimmune phenomena and immunotherapy in individuals receiving long-term benefit.[16, 17]

Similarly, the weight played by environmental factors is clearly demonstrated in the field of autoimmunity, for example by the relatively discordant penetrance in idenetical twins of phenotypes. The role of environmental factors as determinants of tumor rejection has not been extensively studied, but environmental factors are likely to play a significant role, especially considering the well-described effects of concomitant infections—Cooley's original observations[18]—that started the field of tumor immunology. An important factor that should be included among exogenous modifiers is the heterogeneity of treatments that share a conceptually similar mechanism, such as immune stimulation, but vary quantitatively and qualitatively. This is a salient point to which we will refer later.

The most compelling evidence supporting the role played by the genetic heterogeneity of tumors as a determinant of immune responsiveness resides in the phenomenon of *mixed responders*,[19, 20] the relatively infrequent but well-documented phenomenon characterized by the simultaneously discordant behavior of metastatic lesions in response to the same treatment. In this case, both the genetic background of the host and environmental factors are identical.

We suggest that the mechanisms leading to tumor rejection are multifactorial and encompass all three major categories. As a consequence, understanding these mechanisms in the context of the sometimes uncontrollable nature of human disease will require a systematic collection of samples that cover the variables associated with each of these categories.[13]

The elusive mechanisms of immune rejection

It is perhaps puzzling that after decades of effort the mechanisms responsible for tumor rejection remain elusive. We believe that there are at least three reasons why this goal has yet to be achieved. First, as explained in the previous section, the complexity of the problem requires the simultaneous study of several aspects relevant to TSD. However, most studies have followed a minimalistic approach, analyzing one variable, or at best a few, at a time. This has resulted in the identification of trends, or *modifiers*, that seem to be associated with various aspects of TSD, but yet none has shown strong independent predictive value for the simple reason that none is independently responsible for the phenomenon of TSD. It is likely that TSD and tumor rejection occur when a balance between a myriad of factors that favor elimination of cancer overwhelms an opposing congregation of factors related to the biology of the tumor, or to the host's immune response, that favor tolerance.[13] Thus, two considerations are (1) tumor rejection results from a combination of favorable and unfavorable events, and (2) such combinations may differ among patients and within each patient.

A second limitation to the identification of determinants of tumor rejection is a corollary of the first; the bioinformatics approaches currently used do not apply to the essence of cancer immunebiology. Most observational studies using high-throughput technologies aimed at providing a global view of the phenomenon of immunosurveillance are interpreted through the light of class comparison. This, in turn, is based on the straightforward principle that given two phenotypes (i.e., responder and nonresponder) features will be identified using a univariate comparison approach that can distinguish between them. This approach has worked well for monogenetic diseases such as cystic fibrosis, in which the presence or absence of the mutant linearly corresponds to the occurrence of the phenotype. However, as the complexity of interaction among different factors increases, the likelihood of identifying determinants rapidly decreases because it is not the individual but the combination of factors that matters.[21] This problem is compounded by high stringency criteria that require correction for number of tests. Unrealistically high levels of significance are expected for the acceptance of factors of potential relevance. This approach likely eliminates a significant number of cofactors that could be used in combination to construct the algorithm leading to tumor rejection.

A third limitation is related to the second one. Although biostatisticians invoke larger and larger numbers and smaller and smaller *P* values, the re-

ality of tumor immunology is constrained by the small size of clinical trials, as standard therapy is not practiced and most investigations are limited to phase I or II trials. Larger and less common phase III studies take place, but they are generally run by pharmaceutical companies that have shown little interest in including among the goals of their trials those that do not directly pertain to the licensing of their products.

Understanding tumor rejection

Here, we provide a wide-ranging map for the understanding of the phenomenon of tumor rejection, which confronts the three barriers described by the previous section (Fig. 1). The solution to the first problem is evident: a multifactorial analysis based on biological principles needs to be followed. We have recently shown that the coordinated expression of CXCR3 and CCR5 by T cells used for adoptive transfer bears much higher predictive value upon immune responsiveness than does either one alone. In addition, correction for RNA expression by a polymorphism of the CCR5 gene that predicts lack of functional protein strongly increased the predictive value (Bedognetti *et al.*, unpublished results). This is an example of the need to look at distinct components relevant to a biological phenomenon. Thus, the solution to this problem is to collect material suitable for analysis of germ line, epigenetic, and somatic variables timed according to the phenomenon studied.

The solution to the second problem is more complex. The adoption of nonlinear approaches to the analysis of clinical material faces not only resistance by most bioinformaticians, but it is also daunted by the extraordinary computational power needed for combinatorial approaches. A good example is the previously mentioned example of the coordinate expression of CXCR3 and CCR5, corrected for the CCR5 polymorphism. This combination was considered based on a hypothesis-driven analysis of factors known to be relevant to the ICR. Imagining that this combination needed to be discovered computationally by sorting among thousands of gene expression values and millions of polymorphisms provides perspective and the scale of the problem. We, therefore, suggested a stepwise process.

First, low-stringency class comparison should enrich for potentially relevant entities. This process,

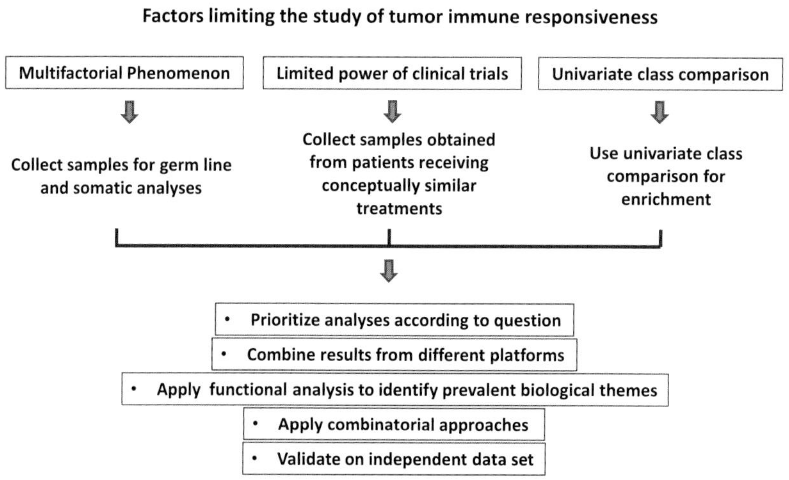

Factors limiting the study of tumor immune responsiveness

Figure 1. Factors limiting the study of tumor-immune responsiveness in humans and a broad-based recipe for the identification of the algorithm governing tumor rejection.

generally referred to as *gene enrichment*, is possibly misleading because in reality this step intends to skim off from the bulk of information entities unlikely to play a role, which therefore reduces the computational power required for further analysis. This process may apply to any platform, including germ line assessment, epigenetics variations, alternation in copy number and gene expression, and protein status.

The second step consists of a functional analysis to identify prominent pathways (here the term *enriched* may apply) according to the entities selected by the first step (in the CXCR3/CCR5 example, the two genes belong to the same functional category and their expression is often concomitant during ICR). Upon identifying predominant pathways, combinatorial analyses could focus on each individual, thus alleviating the computational burden. Probabilistic logic methods of this kind have been unpopular in clinical research, but they should be applied in the future.[22]

The limited number of patients enrolled in immunotherapy trials could be overcome by assessing cases congregated according to conceptually similar therapeutic modalities considered as a single exogenous environmental factor. Thus, the genetic makeup of the host and tumor cells would function as independent variables similarly interacting with exogenous entities. And while genetic determinants idiosyncratic to individual treatment may be missed by this approach, the salient components

determining the emergence of the conserved ICR phenomenon will emerge.

Summary

Here, we have described a broad-based approach to understanding the phenomenon of tumor rejection in humans, an approach that covers three major categories likely to be involved. We predict that by following this forensic approach, which systematically balances hypothesis and discovery, an algorithm will be uncovered that governs TSD by activation of the immunological constant of rejection.

Acknowledgments

The authors would like to acknowledge the Hasumi Foundation for organizing the 7th International Cancer Vaccine Symposium and all of the participants who, with their expertise, greatly improved the development of this paper.

Conflicts of interest

The authors declare no conflicts of interest.

References

1. Shankaran, V., H. Ikeda, A.T. Bruce, *et al.* 2001. IFN-g and lymphocytes prevent primary tumour development and shape tumour immunogenicity. *Nature* **410:** 1107–1111.
2. Dunn, G.P., A.T. Bruce, H. Ikeda, *et al.* 2002. Cancer immunoediting: from immunosurveillance to tumor escape. *Nature Immunol.* **3:** 991–998.
3. Burnet, F.M. 1970. The concept of immunological surveillance. *Prog. Exp. Tumor. Res.* **13:** 1–27.

4. Galon, J., A. Costes, F. Sanchez-Cabo, *et al.* 2006. Type, density, and location of immune cells within human colorectal tumors predict clinical outcome. *Science* **313:** 1960–1964.

5. Ascierto, M.L., V. De Giorgi, Q. Liu, *et al.* 2011. An immunologic portrait of cancer. *J. Transl. Med.* **9:** 146.

6. Louahed, J., O. Grusell, S. Gaulis, *et al.* 2008. Expression of defined genes indentifed by pre-treatment tumor profiling: association with clinical response to GSK MAGE A-3 immunetherapeutic in metastatic melanoma patients. *J. Clin. Oncol.* **26:** A9045.

7. Gajewski, T.F., J. Louahed & V.G. Brichard. 2010. Gene signature in melanoma associated with clinical activity: a potential clue to unlock cancer immunotherapy. *Cancer J.* **16:** 399–403.

8. Wang, E., A. Worschech & F.M. Marincola. 2008. The immunologic constant of rejection. *Trends Immunol.* **29:** 256–262.

9. Sarwal, M., M.S. Chua, N. Kambham, *et al.* 2003. Molecular heterogeneity in acute renal allograft rejection identified by DNA microarray profiling. *N. Engl. J. Med.* **349:** 125–138.

10. Imanguli, M.M., W.D. Swaim, S.C. League, *et al.* 2009. Increased T-bet+ cytotoxic effectors and type I interferon-mediated processes in chronic graft-versus-host disease of the oral mucosa. *Blood* **113:** 3620–3630.

11. Dunn, G.P., L.J. Old & R.D. Schreiber. 2004. The three Es of cancer immunoediting. *Annu. Rev. Immunol.* **22:** 329–360.

12. Wang, E., L.D. Miller, G.A. Ohnmacht, *et al.* 2002. Prospective molecular profiling of subcutaneous melanoma metastases suggests classifiers of immune responsiveness. *Cancer Res.* **62:** 3581–3586.

13. Wang, E., S. Tomei & F.M. Marincola. 2012. Reflections upon human cancer immune responsiveness to T cell-based therapy. *Cancer Immunol. Immunother.* **61:** 761–770.

14. Sestak, A.L., B.G. Fürnrohr, J.B. Harley, *et al.* 2011. The genetics of systemic lupus erythematosus and implications for targeted therapy. *Ann. Rheum. Dis.* **70**(Suppl. 1): i37–i43.

15. Uccellini, L., V. De Giorgi, Y. Zhao, *et al.* 2012. IRF5 gene polymorphisms in melanoma. *J. Transl. Med.* **10:** 170.

16. Phan, G.Q., P. Attia, S.M. Steinberg, *et al.* 2001. Factors associated with response to high-dose interleukin-2 in patients with metastatic melanoma. *J. Clin. Oncol.* **19:** 3477–3482.

17. Gogas, H., J. Ioannovich, U. Dafni, *et al.* 2006. Prognostic significance of autoimmunity during treatment of melanoma with interferon. *N. Engl. J. Med.* **354:** 709–718.

18. Old, L.J. 1996. Immunotherapy for cancer. *Sci. Am.* **275:** 136–143.

19. Bornhauser, M., U. Klenk, C. Rollig, *et al.* 2004. Mixed response after allogeneic haemopoietic-cell transplantation for metastatic renal-cell carcinoma. *Lancet Oncol.* **5:** 191–192.

20. Carretero, R., E. Wang, A.I. Rodriguez, *et al.* 2012. Regression of melanoma metastases after immunotherapy is associated with activation of antigen presentation and interferon-mediated rejection genes. *Int. J. Cancer* **131:** 387–395.

21. Han, B., X.W. Chen, Z. Talebizadeh & H. Xu. 2012. Genetic studies of complex human diseases: characterizing SNP-disease associations using Bayesian networks. *BMC Syst. Biol.* **6**(Suppl. 3): S14.

22. Sakhanenko, N.A. & D.J. Galas. 2012. Probabilistic logic methods and some applications to biology and medicine. *J. Comput. Biol.* **19:** 316–336.

Ann. N.Y. Acad. Sci. ISSN 0077-8923

ANNALS OF THE NEW YORK ACADEMY OF SCIENCES

Issue: *The Renaissance of Cancer Immunotherapy*

Cancer-induced immunosuppressive cascades and their reversal by molecular-targeted therapy

Yutaka Kawakami, Tomonori Yaguchi, Hidetoshi Sumimoto, Chie Kudo-Saito, Nobuo Tsukamoto, Tomoko Iwata-Kajihara, Shoko Nakamura, Hiroshi Nishio, Ryosuke Satomi, Asuka Kobayashi, Mayuri Tanaka, Jeong Hoon Park, Hajime Kamijuku, Takahiro Tsujikawa, and Naoshi Kawamura

Division of Cellular Signaling, Institute for Advanced Medical Research, Keio University School of Medicine, Tokyo, Japan

Address for correspondence: Yutaka Kawakami, Division of Cellular Signaling, Institute for Advanced Medical Research, Keio University School of Medicine, 35 Shinanomachi, Shinjuku, Tokyo, Japan. yutakawa@z5.keio.jp

Immunological status in tumor tissues varies among patients. Infiltration of memory-type CD8$^+$ T cells into tumors correlates with prognosis of patients with various cancers. However, the mechanism of the differential CD8$^+$ T cell infiltration has not been well investigated. In general, tumor-associated microenvironments, including tumor and sentinel lymph nodes, are under immunosuppressive conditions such that the immune system is not able to eliminate cancer cells without immune-activating interventions. Constitutive activation of various signaling pathways in human cancer cells triggers multiple immunosuppressive cascades that involve various cytokines, chemokines, and immunosuppressive cells. Signaling pathway inhibitors could inhibit these immunosuppressive cascades by acting on either cancer or immune cells, or both. In addition, common signaling mechanisms are often utilized for multiple hallmarks of cancer (e.g., cell proliferation/survival, invasion/metastasis, and immunosuppression). Therefore, targeting these common signaling pathways may be an attractive strategy for cancer therapy including immunotherapy.

Keywords: immunosuppression; BRAF; STAT3; β-catenin; NF-κB

Introduction

Human tumor antigens recognized by T cells have previously been identified in our studies and applied to various cancer immunotherapies.[1,2] One such melanoma antigen, gp100, was isolated by cDNA expression cloning using tumor infiltrating T cells (TILs).[3–6] In a recent multicenter, randomized clinical trial, gp100 peptide vaccination combined with interleukin 2 (IL-2) resulted in a 16% objective response with 9% complete response (CR).[7] In contrast, adoptive immunotherapy using cultured TILs following myelo-lymphoablative treatment, which depletes various immunosuppressive cells, resulted in more than 70% objective response with 20% durable CR in advanced melanoma patients with multiple metastases.[8] These studies indicate that immunosuppressive conditions, particularly in tumor-associated microenviron-ments such as tumor and sentinel lymph nodes (SLNs), are one of the major obstacles for the development of effective immunotherapy. Thus, understanding the mechanisms of cancer cell–induced immunosuppression in tumor-associated microenvironments and developing methods to reverse immunosuppression are important for immunotherapy.

Tumor-associated microenvironments

During cancer development, cancer cells, various immune cells, and other stromal cells, such as fibroblasts and mesenchymal stem cells, interact, and immunoediting via immunosurveillance and immunoescape defines immunological characteristics of cancer cells (e.g., loss of highly immunogenic tumor antigens, acquirement of resistance to immune cells, and ability to suppress immune response).[9] Thus, cancer cells seen in the clinic are generally

doi: 10.1111/nyas.12094

Ann. N.Y. Acad. Sci. 1284 (2013) 80–86 © 2013 New York Academy of Sciences.

immunosuppressive and generate immunosuppressive conditions in tumor-associated microenvironments. Immunosuppressive cells, such as myeloid-derived suppressor cells (MDSCs) and regulatory T (T$_{reg}$) cells, are increased, while dendritic cells (DCs) appear to be impaired in tumors and sentinel lymph nodes in cancer patients.[10] Interestingly, immune status varies among patients, as reflected by recent findings showing that the level of infiltration of memory CD8$^+$ T cells in tumors differs among cancer patients. More CD8$^+$ T cell infiltration correlated with favorable prognosis in various cancers, including colon and ovarian cancer, and also correlated with the response to immunotherapy or chemotherapy in patients with melanoma or colon cancer, respectively.[11, 12] However, the mechanisms underlying differences in immune status among cancer patients remain to be investigated.

Gene and signaling alterations in cancer cells

Immune status in tumor microenvironments may be regulated by stimulating factors for antitumor immune response, including expression of immunogenic tumor antigens and human leukocyte antigen (HLA), spontaneous immune response cascades (such as the pathway from tumor DNA to IFN-producing DCs to CD8$^+$ T cell induction),[13] or by immunosuppressive cytokines such as transforming growth factor β (TGF-β) and IL-10. Since TGF-β is produced by most cancer cells and some infiltrating immune and stromal cells, we have evaluated the role of TGF-β in tumor microenvironments. In a mouse tumor model, increased TGF-β expression in tumor microenvironments via implantation of TGF-β cDNA–transfected tumor cells resulted in increased infiltration of immunosuppressive CD11b$^+$ Gr-1$^+$ MDSCs and FoxP3$^+$ CD4$^+$ T$_{reg}$ cells in both tumors and SLNs. Infiltration of DCs was decreased in tumors; in SLNs the number of DCs was increased compared to non-SLNs in mice with either TGF-β–transduced or mock-transduced tumor cells, but T cell stimulatory activity of DCs was significantly impaired in mice with TGF-β$^+$ tumors. M2-like macrophages producing abundant CCL22, which recruits CCR4$^+$ T$_{reg}$ and Th2 cells, were also increased in both tumors and SLNs.[14] Consequently, induction of tumor-specific T cells in SLNs was significantly reduced, which probably led to decreased infiltration

of CD8$^+$ T cells in tumors. Therefore, the mouse tumor model recapitulates some of the immune conditions in tumors and SLNs in cancer patients (work in progress). An increase in immunosuppressive factors such as TGF-β may be one of the mechanisms defining the immune status of tumor microenvironments, such as spontaneous CD8$^+$ T cell responses.

We have also found that the TGF-β-induced transcription factor, Snail, which is known to promote metastasis via epithelial-to-mesenchymal transition (EMT) in cancer cells, also enhances production of multiple immunosuppressive cytokines and chemokines, including TGF-β, IL-10, CCL2, and TSP-1, which cause DC impairment and T$_{reg}$ cell induction. The impaired DCs have less T cell stimulatory activity and induce T$_{reg}$ cells. CCL2 not only impairs DC function but also recruits MDSCs into tumors. Intratumoral administration of Snail-specific siRNA restored immunocompetence of mice implanted with Snail-expressing tumor, and resulted in induction of tumor antigen–specific T cells.[15]

In a more recent work in progress, we have identified an upstream signaling molecule of TGF-β production in human cancer cells by screening immunosuppressive activity in DCs using a kinase siRNA library (unpublished data). The identified kinase is significantly phosphorylated in human cancer cells, and its depletion suppressed TGF-β production by cancer cells (manuscript in preparation). These results indicate that TGF-β, produced by either cancer cells or infiltrated stromal cells in tumor microenvironments, triggers immunosuppressive cascades involving various immunosuppressive cytokines, chemokines, and cells, and reemphasizes that TGF-β cascade is an attractive target for reversal of cancer-induced immunosuppression (Fig. 1).

Multiple immunosuppressive cascades in human cancers

Gene and signal alterations in human cancer cells vary among cancer types, and even within the same type of cancer. Therefore, we have evaluated immunosuppressive mechanisms of various human cancers (Fig. 1).

MAPK signal pathway

We have found that activation of the mitogen-activated protein kinase (MAPK) signal pathway via common BRAF mutation (V600E) not only

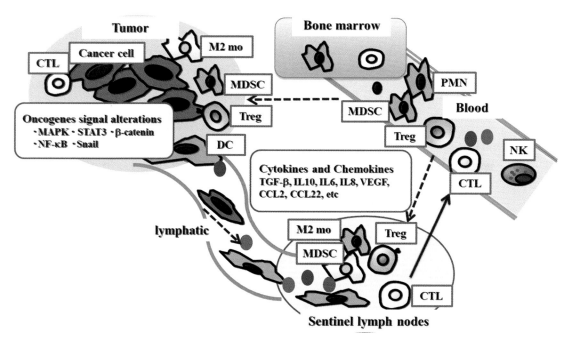

Figure 1. Alterations of genes and signaling in cancer cells trigger multiple immunosuppressive cascades. Alterations of oncogenes and subsequently activated signaling, such as MAPK, STAT3, β-catenin, and NF-κB in human cancer cells, trigger multiple immunosuppressive cascades, including production of multiple immunosuppressive cytokines and chemokines, such as TGF-β, IL-10, CCL2, subsequent impairment of DC function, and induction of various immunosuppressive cells such as MDSCs, M2-like macrophages, and T_{reg} cells.

promotes melanoma cell proliferation and invasion but also promotes production of multiple immunosuppressive cytokines, such as IL-6, IL-10, and VEGF.[16,17] These cytokines suppress T cell stimulatory activity of DCs through decreased IL-12 and TNF-α production and increased IL-10 production. Treatment of human melanoma cells with BRAF (V600E)-specific shRNA or MEK inhibitors resulted in decreased immunosuppressive activity, indicating that the MAPK pathway is involved in DC impairment by melanoma cells.[17] Therefore, the BRAF–MAPK axis is involved in multiple hallmarks of cancer, including cancer cell proliferation, invasion, and immunosuppression. Blockade of the BRAF–MAPK axis not only inhibits cell proliferation and invasion of, but also reverses immunosuppression by melanoma cells, indicating that the MAPK signal pathway might be an attractive target for melanoma treatment (Fig. 2).[16,17]

Although MAPK inhibition may also suppress proliferation of antitumor T cells, recently developed BRAF inhibitors that preferentially inhibit mutant BRAF may have less T cell inhibitory activity.

In clinical trials, administration of BRAF inhibitors reduced tumor size in some patients, indicating induction of melanoma cell death *in vivo.*[18] Therefore, the selective mutant BRAF inhibitors may be useful in combination with immunotherapies through the following mechanisms: (1) reduction of tumor volume via cell death and inhibition of proliferation, subsequent decrease of immunosuppressive activity, and increased release of endogenous tumor antigens, including unique mutated antigens, leading to induction of multiple autologous tumor-specific T cells due to less inhibitory activity of the selective BRAF inhibitors for T cell proliferation; (2) restoration of immunocompetence via decreased production of multiple immunosuppressive cytokines, and subsequent simultaneous inhibition of multiple immunosuppressive cascades; (3) increased susceptibility of melanoma cells to cytotoxic T cells (CTLs) due to the reported increased expression of melanosomal tumor antigens;[19] and (4) decreased metastatic ability of melanoma cells. In fact, administration of mutant BRAF–selective inhibitor alone has recently demonstrated increased

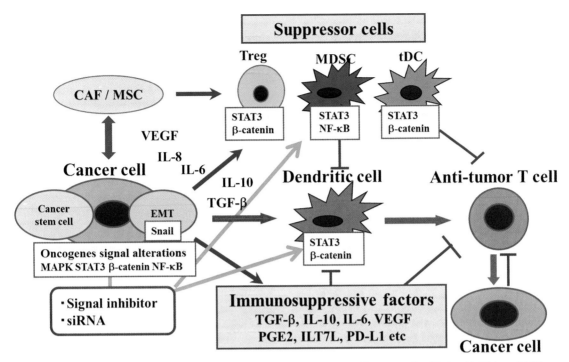

Figure 2. Reversal of cancer-induced immunosuppression by targeting cancer and immune cells with signal inhibitors. Inhibitors for altered signaling molecules, such as BRAF, STAT3, β-catenin, and NF-κB, may restore immunocompetence of cancer patients by acting on both cancer cells and various immune cells, such as DCs, MDSCs, and T_{reg} cells.

infiltration of granzyme-positive CD8$^+$ T cells in tumors, which correlated with tumor reduction.[20]

STAT3 signal pathway

Activation of STAT3 signaling is also observed in human melanoma cells. Similar to BRAF depletion, STAT3 depletion by lentiviral shRNA resulted in inhibition of multiple immunosuppressive cytokines, including IL-6, IL-10, and VEGF.[17] These cytokines activate STAT3 in various immune cells, including DCs, MDSCs, and T_{reg} cells, rendering them immunosuppressive. In a mouse tumor model, STAT3-depleted DCs were found to be resistant to tumor-derived immunosuppressive factors and to have enhanced T cell stimulatory activity via high IL-12 production.[21] Injection of STAT3-depleted DCs into tumors that are immunosuppressed resulted in stronger antitumor effects accompanied by induction of IFN-γ–producing tumor-specific T cells compared to regular DCs.[21] Similarly, subsequent work in progress has indicated that STAT3-depleted macrophages are also resistant to tumor-derived immunosuppressive cytokines, and induction of immunosuppressive MDSCs expressing arginase may

be inhibited by STAT3 depletion. These results indicate that activation of STAT3 in cancer cells triggers induction of various immunosuppressive cells, including tolerogenic DCs and MDSCs, partly via STAT3 activation in the immune cells. Therefore, STAT3 inhibitors may also be useful for reversal of cancer-induced immunosuppression by acting on both cancer cells and various immune cells.

In a murine tumor model, various STAT3 inhibitors have been shown to augment antitumor immunity.[22,23] STAT3 inhibitors are currently being evaluated as cancer therapy in clinical trials, and their immunological effects should be evaluated in the future. In addition, inhibitors of upstream molecules of STAT3, including JAK and further upstream molecules such as EGF-R/VEGF-R, are already available in clinic, and may be useful for reversal of immunosuppression and combined use with immunotherapy. JAK inhibitors have been shown to augment antitumor immunity and enhance antitumor effects in combination with immunotherapies, such as IL-12 administration.[24] We have preliminary data indicating that EGF-R inhibitors can suppress production of immunosuppressive cytokines from human lung cancer cells with EGF-R mutations; administration of EGF-R inhibitors along with cancer vaccines seems to provide synergistic antitumor effects through direct and indirect enhancement of T cell stimulatory activity of DCs in murine tumor models (the indirect enhancement may be via decreased immunosuppressive cytokines from cancer cells). Administration of a multikinase inhibitor, sunitinib, which also suppresses downstream STAT3 signaling, was reported to decrease MDSCs and T$_{reg}$ cells, and increase IFN-γ–producing T cells, in renal cell carcinoma (RCC) patients.[25] Administration of dasatinib, another multikinase inhibitor that also inhibits downstream STAT3 signaling, resulted in increased response rates in some patients with Ph1$^+$ CML and ALL, accompanied by LGL lymphocytosis- and autoimmune-like syndrome.[26] In other work in progress and thus far unpublished, we have found natural compounds in traditional Japanese Kampo medicines that inhibit STAT3 and MAPK pathways, as well as augment antitumor T cell responses when administered in murine tumor models. These observations are consistent with the idea that STAT3 inhibition strategies may be useful for immunotherapy.

NF-κB signal pathway

Some human ovarian cancers produce high amounts of IL-6, IL-8, and CCL2 in a NF-κB–dependent manner. In unpublished preliminary studies, we have found that high plasma levels of IL-6 and IL-8 correlated with poor prognosis of cancer patients and poor response to various immunotherapies. NF-κB inhibitor not only inhibited production of IL-6, IL-8, and CCL2 by cancer cells, but also inhibited differentiation of monocytes to immunosuppressive macrophages in the presence of cancer cell–derived factors. Administration of the NF-κB inhibitor enhanced antitumor T cell responses possibly through reversal of immunosuppressive conditions in a murine tumor model (manuscript in preparation). In human RCC, an NF-κB inhibitor was also found to decrease the intrinsic expression of ILT7L, which inhibits IFN-α production by plasmacytoid DCs.[27] These results indicate that appropriate doses of NF-κB inhibitors may augment antitumor T cell responses by acting on both cancer and immune cells, although high doses of NF-κB inhibitors may also ameliorate induction of antitumor T cells.

Wnt/β-catenin signal pathway

Activation of the Wnt/β-catenin pathway is observed in about 30% of human melanomas and correlates with IL-10 production by melanoma cells. Culture supernatant of melanoma cells generated DCs with high IL-10 and low IL-12 production, less T cell stimulatory activity *in vitro* (partly in an IL-10–dependent manner), and an ability to induce FOXP3$^+$ T$_{reg}$ cells. Pretreatment of melanoma cells with β-catenin-shRNA reduced these immunosuppressive activities. When the β–catenin-activated human melanoma cells were implanted in severe combined immunodeficiency (SCID) mice, mouse DCs in spleen and tumor had impaired T cell stimulatory activity, partly due to IL-10 produced by human melanoma cells.[28] Administration of a β-catenin inhibitor restored the T cell stimulatory activity in splenic DCs of these mice.[28] Since β-catenin was reported to be involved in generation of regulatory DCs and survival of T$_{reg}$, β-catenin inhibitor may also be useful for reversal of cancer-induced immunosuppression by acting on both cancer and immune cells.

Clinical implications of immunosuppression mechanisms

The specific steps that should be inhibited in these immunosuppressive cascades for effective reversal of immunosuppression in cancer patients have yet to be identified.[10] Targeting activated signaling molecules in cancer cells, upstream of the cascades, may simultaneously inhibit multiple immunosuppressive mechanisms and exert direct antitumor effects, such as inhibition of cancer cell proliferation and destruction of cancer cells, which may lead to further induction of immune responses to endogenous tumor antigens, including patients' unique antigens (e.g., mutated antigens). Signal inhibitors may also have direct effects on immune cells, including direct activation of immune cells or inhibition of generation of immunosuppressive cells, such as T$_{reg}$ cells and MDSCs (Fig. 2). However, upstream inhibition may also cause more broad adverse effects, including suppression of antitumor immune response; although it may be avoided by use of appropriate doses of inhibitors, as shown for NF-κB inhibitor, or by use of mutant molecule-specific inhibitors, such as mutant BRAF-selective inhibitors. In contrast, downstream targeting, including of immunosuppressive effectors such as TGF-β, IL-10,

PD-L1, IDO, Cox2, MDSCs, and T_{reg} cells, by using antibodies or small molecule inhibitors may result in more specific and efficient blockade with less broad adverse effects, although inhibition of one molecule or cell type may be insufficient to reverse immunosuppression overall. The combination of upstream signal inhibitors and downstream blockade of major immuosuppressive factors (e.g., neutralizing or blocking Ab for TGF-β and PD-L1) may also be an attractive strategy for effective restoration of antitumor immune responses.

Altogether, targeting activated signaling molecules involved in triggering multiple immunosuppressive cascades may effectively treat cancer through restoration of antitumor immune responses. Combined treatment with these molecular-targeted drugs and various immunotherapies, including cancer vaccines and check point blockade, should be evaluated in future clinical trials. Since activated signaling molecules are different among patients even with the same type of cancers, using personalized strategies will be important. In addition to their therapeutic implications, evaluation of altered gene/signaling status (e.g., pERK, pSTAT3, nuclear translocation of NF-κB, or β-catenin) may also be useful for diagnosis of cancer patients because altered gene and signaling affect immune status, indicated by, for example, tumor infiltration of memory $CD8^+$ T cells and level of serum cytokines (e.g., IL-6, IL-8), which correlates with prognosis and treatment response in cancer patients.

Conclusion

Understanding the molecular basis of immunopathology in tumor-associated microenvironments is essential for the development of effective cancer diagnostic methods and therapy, not only for immunotherapy, but also for other standard cancer therapies such as chemotherapy. In particular, immunotherapy (e.g., cancer vaccine and check point blockade) combined with molecular-targeted drugs, currently used as single agents, is a promising strategy to be exploited in future clinical trials.

Acknowledgments

The authors thank Ms. Misako Horikawa and Ms. Ryoko Suzuki for assistance with manuscript preparation. This work was supported by Grants-in-Aid for Scientific Research (23240128, 21591445) from the Japan Society for Promotion of Science, a research program of the Project for Development of Innovative Research on Cancer Therapeutics (P-Direct) from the Ministry of Education, Culture, Sports, Science and Technology, a Grant-in-Aid for Cancer Research from the Ministry of Health, Labor and Welfare, and Translational Research grant from New Energy and Industrial Technology Development Organization, Japan.

Conflicts of interest

The authors declare no conflicts of interest.

References

1. Kawakami, Y., T. Fujita, Y. Matsuzaki, *et al.* 2004. Identification of human tumor antigens and its implications for diagnosis and treatment of cancer. *Cancer Sci.* **95**: 784–791.
2. Kawakami, Y., S. Eliyahu, C.H. Delgado, *et al.* 1994. Cloning of the gene coding for a shared human melanoma antigen recognized by autologous T cells infiltrating into tumor. *Proc. Natl. Acad. Sci. U.S.A.* **91**: 3515–1519.
3. Kawakami, Y., S. Eliyahu, C.H. Delgado, *et al.* 1994. Identification of human melanoma antigen recognized by tumor infiltrating lymphocytes associated with in vivo tumor rejection. *Proc. Natl. Acad. Sci. U.S.A.* **91**: 6458–6462.
4. Kawakami, Y., S. Eliyafu & C. Jennings. 1995. Recognition of multiple epitopes in the human melanoma antigens gp100 by tumor infiltrating T-lymphocytes associated with in vivo tumor regression. *J. Immunol.* **154**: 3961–3968.
5. Parkhurst, M.R., M.L. Salgaller, S. Southwood, *et al.* 1996. Improved induction of melanoma reactive CTL with peptides from the melanoma antigen gp100 modified at HLA-A*0201 binding residues. *J. Immunol.* **157**: 2539–2548.
6. Rosenberg, S.A., J. Yang, D. Schwartzentruber, *et al.* 1998. Immunologic and therapeutic evaluation of a synthetic peptide vaccine for the treatment of patients with metastatic melanoma. *Nat. Med.* **4**: 321–327.
7. Schwartzentruber, D.J., D.H. Lawson, J.M. Richards, *et al.* 2011. gp100 peptide vaccine and interleukin-2 in patients with advanced melanoma. *N. Engl. J. Med.* **364**: 2119–2127.
8. Rosenberg, S.A., J.C. Yang, R.M. Sherry, *et al.* 2011. Durable complete responses in heavily pretreated patients with metastatic melanoma using T-cell transfer immunotherapy. *Clin. Cancer Res.* **17**: 4550–4557.
9. Schreiber, R.D., L.J. Old & M.J. Smyth. 2011. Cancer immunoediting: integrating immunity's roles in cancer suppression and promotion. *Science* **331**: 1565–1570.
10. Yaguchi, T., H. Sumimoto, C. Kudo-Saito, *et al.* 2011. The mechanisms of cancer immunoescape and development of overcoming strategies. *Int. J. Hematol.* **93**: 294–300.
11. Fridman, W.H., F. Pagès, C. Sautès-Fridman & J. Galon. 2012. The immune contexture in human tumours: impact on clinical outcome. *Nat. Rev. Cancer* **12**: 298–306.
12. Galon, J., F. Pagès, F.M. Marincola, *et al.* 2012. Cancer classification using the immunoscore: a worldwide task force. *J. Transl. Med.* **10**: 205.

13. Fuertes, M.B., S.R. Woo, B. Burnett, *et al.* 2013. Type I interferon response and innate immune sensing of cancer. *Trends Immunol.* **34:** 67–73.

14. Tsujikawa, T., T. Yaguchi, G. Ohmura, *et al.* 2013. Autocrine and paracrine loops between cancer cells and macrophages promote lymph node metastasis via CCR4/CCL22 in head and neck squamous cell carcinoma. *Int. J. Cancer.* DOI: 10.1002/ijc.27966.

15. Kudo-Saito, C., H. Shirako, T. Takeuchi & Y. Kawakami. 2009. Cancer metastasis is accelerated through immunosuppression during Snail-induced EMT of cancer cells. *Cancer Cell* **15:** 195–206.

16. Sumimoto, H., M. Miyagishi, H. Miyoshi, *et al.* 2004. Inhibition of growth and invasive ability of melanoma by inactivation of mutated BRAF with lentivirus-mediated RNA interference. *Oncogene* **23:** 6031–6039.

17. Sumimoto, H., F. Imabayashi, T. Iwata & Y. Kawakami. 2006. The BRAF-MAPK signaling pathway is essential for cancer-immune evasion in human melanoma cells. *J. Exp. Med.* **203:** 1651–1656.

18. Chapman, P.B., A. Hauschild, C. Robert, *et al.* 2011. Improved survival with vemurafenib in melanoma with BRAF V600E mutation. *N. Engl. J. Med.* **364:** 2507–2516.

19. Boni, A., A.P. Cogdill, P. Dang, *et al.* 2010. Selective BRAFV600E inhibition enhances T-cell recognition of melanoma without affecting lymphocyte function. *Cancer Res.* **70:** 5213–5219.

20. Wilmott, J.S., G.V. Long, J.R. Howle, *et al.* 2011. Selective BRAF inhibitors induce marked T-cell infiltration into human metastatic melanoma. *Clin. Cancer Res.* **18:** 1386–1394.

21. Iwata-Kajihara, T., H. Sumimoto, N. Kawamura, *et al.* 2011. Enhanced cancer immunotherapy using STAT3-depleted dendritic cells with high Th1-inducing ability and resistance to cancer cell-derived inhibitory factors. *J. Immunol.* **187:** 27–36.

22. Kortylewski, M., M. Kujawski, T. Wang, *et al.* 2005. Inhibiting Stat3 signaling in the hematopoietic system elicits multi-component antitumor immunity. *Nat. Med.* **11:** 1314–1321.

23. Lee, H., S.K. Pal, K. Reckamp, *et al.* 2011. STAT3: a target to enhance antitumor immune response. *Curr. Top. Microbiol. Immunol.* **344:** 41–59.

24. Burdelya, L., R. Catlett-Falcone, A. Levitzki, *et al.* 2002. Combination therapy with AG-490 and interleukin 12 achieves greater antitumor effects than either agent alone. *Mol. Cancer Ther.* **1:** 893–899.

25. Ko, J.S., A.H. Zea, B.I. Rini, *et al.* 2009. Sunitinib mediates reversal of myeloid-derived suppressor cell accumulation in renal cell carcinoma patients. *Clin. Cancer Res.* **15:** 2148–2157.

26. Mustjoki, S., M. Ekblom, T.P. Arstila, *et al.* 2009. Clonal expansion of T/NK-cells during tyrosine kinase inhibitor dasatinib therapy. *Leukemia* **23:** 1398–1405.

27. Tsukamoto, N., S. Okada, Y. Onami, *et al.* 2009. Impairment of plasmacytoid dendritic cells for IFN production by the ligand for immunoglobulin-like transcript 7 expressed on human cancer cells. *Clin. Cancer Res.* **15:** 5733–5743.

28. Yaguchi, T., Y. Goto, K. Kido, *et al.* 2012. Immune suppression and resistance mediated by constitutive activation of Wnt/β-catenin signaling in human melanoma cells. *J. Immunol.* **189:** 2110–2117.